SHAPE UP FOR SPORTS

SHAPE UP FOR SPORTS

by RAY SIEGENER

A BERKLEY WINDHOVER BOOK
published by
BERKLEY PUBLISHING CORPORATION

Acknowledgments

I would like to express my appreciation to some special people in sports who have advised or encouraged me in pursuit of this project or who have contributed in some way to SHAPE UP FOR SPORTS. They include: Earl Monroe, Frank Gifford, Laura Baugh, Billie Jean King, Roy White, George Blanda, Suzy Chaffee, Tug McGraw, Dick Keelor, Kyle Rote, Jr., Dr. George Sheehan, Gary Wiren, and the New York Knick's Danny Whalen. Thanks to The Gym in New York for the use of their facilities for photography. And thanks to Harry D. Kaufman for his Swedish Walking Program.

Acknowledgment is made to *Runner's World* Magazine for Dr. Sheehan's words on foot injuries which appeared in "Booklet of the Month" number 1, 1971. A thank you to Joseph Zohar, R.P.T. for his excellent tennis exercises. The section on weight training for women was reprinted by permission of *WomenSports* Magazine, January, 1975. Gary Wiren's program for golfers was reprinted courtesy of *Golf Digest* Magazine from the December, 1974 issue, copyright Golf Digest, Inc., 1974. "Danger Signs and What to Do About Them" was adapted from *Exercise Your Way to Fitness and Health* by Lenore Zohman, M.D., 1974. The "Intermediate Jogging Program" is reprinted from U.S. Department of Agriculture Publication No. 7661 2811, *Fitness and Work Capacity* by Brian Sharkey. The following sections were edited by the author for the *Conditioning for a Purpose* series and are reprinted herein with the permission of the National Varsity Club: Baseball by Roy White, Basketball by Gale Goodrich, Football by Roger Staubach, Distance Running by

Jim Ryun, Soccer by Gordon Bradley, Swimming by Jack Nelson, Tennis by Jimmy Connors and Stan Smith, Wrestling by Dan Gable, and Running Tips by Paul Warfield.

The Travelers Insurance Companies get a vote of thanks for allowing me to use the text and photos from the strength portion of their program *Conditioning for Fire Fighters.*

And very special thanks to my typist Kathleen Judge; my wife, Julia and the troops, Raymond, Susan and Kristin for putting up with all the hassles of another book; and to my editor, Robin Rosenthal.

Contents

PREFACE

When I set out to write this book, its purpose was quite clear and straightforward. As the title indicates, the book is intended to be a manual for those who enjoy or hope to enjoy recreational sports. After being involved for several years with many of the country's leading athletes and coaches and the President's Council on Physical Fitness and Sports in the preparation of training and motivation materials for young athletes, I shifted my focus to the weekend athlete. It was obvious that the person who indulges in sports for fun needs help in terms of adequate conditioning and the avoidance of injury.

My research for this project required me to seek out my many friends in sports in order to get a solid perspective on how professional athletes perceive their fitness and conditioning activities and what advice they might have for my readers. I was looking for the best possible programs—activities that would help the weekend athlete develop his sports fitness: endurance, strength and flexibility. These had to be realistic programs that would allow a person to start at ground zero and progress to the desired level of fitness for his or her sport.

Richard O. Keelor, Ph.D., the Director of Program Development for the President's Council on Physical Fitness and Sports, a friend and valued adviser, helped me to find the exercise routines that would be appropriate for the greatest number of people in the weekend-athlete category. It was necessary to provide athletes at many levels of development information with which to build a solid fitness base.

The road to personal fitness has not been an especially well-traveled one in America.

SHAPE UP FOR SPORTS

Recently, though, more of us are trying to travel that road and find it riddled with "potholes" of potential disaster and laced with intriguing detours leading nowhere. Physical-fitness programs fail far too frequently. The inconsistency of the human machine is the villain here. One man's excursion into physical nirvana is another's orthopedic nightmare. Pain, exhaustion, disappointment are too often the lot of the neophyte who dips his or her toe into the sports-fitness maelstrom.

Meanwhile, happily jogging down his own road toward his personal outer limits is a gangly, sinewy, iconoclastic physician from Red Bank, New Jersey. "Fifty-eight years old and growing" is how cardiologist George Sheehan describes himself. Dr. Sheehan is quoted frequently in this book; in fact, he provided me with much useful information regarding the avoidance of sports injuries. But the greatest service Dr. Sheehan has performed for me hits a lot closer to home. George Sheehan helped me to shift gears in terms of my understanding of fitness and its relationship to sports and what both of them are all about.

Dr. Sheehan began running at the age of forty-five. He now runs the Boston annually and every other marathon in sight. He holds the World's Record for the mile for people over fifty. But more important for him and the people he comes into contact with is that he "has returned to his body" and he can make that an exciting concept to his listeners and readers. "We are too serious," he says. "Even when we participate in sports, it's serious. We do it for the wrong reasons. We've got to get play back into our lives. Our sport must be a joyful thing. This means finding the sport that's right for you; so you'll feel as good when you're doing it as I feel when I'm running."

Suzy Chaffee, former Olympic skier, a World Champion free-style skier, admits to being a "soul-sister to Dr. Sheehan." Suzy became intellectually aware of physical fitness after the 1968 Olympics. She found that she missed the energy and the "dynamic feeling of readiness" that her training regimen provided. Since then, Suzy Chaffee's fitness program, which consists of running, gymnastics, ballet, weight training, yoga and cycling, has become a spiritual symbiosis of mind and body. She, too, speaks of the *joy* of physical activity, when the body is prepared for it.

So, thanks to my friends and consultants, Dick Keelor, George Sheehan and Suzy Chaffee, *Shape Up for Sports* is more than a fitness manual for the weekend athlete. It is, unembarrassingly, a sell piece for sport and fitness. It is an exhortation to experience the joy, the sensual trip, of sports; it is an invitation to—"return to your body."

INTRODUCTION

During my years of association with the space program and the government's national fitness effort, I've observed a growing awareness of the need for fitness and physical activity. Perhaps, to use the word *awareness* is to understate the situation. Today, people want to be active. They want to use their bodies as healthy human beings were meant to use them. They want to run and play and sweat a little.

One of the major frustrations that physical educators have had to deal with in the past was the idea that Americans were a nation of spectators. Sports involvement, to many people, meant buying a ticket to a baseball or football game, sitting in the stands, and watching someone else play. Fortunately, this perception of sports has begun to change. George Leonard, in his book *The Ultimate Athlete*, insists that there is an athlete in each of us. To call forth that hidden dimension of ourselves and develop it can be infinitely rewarding.

This book, *Shape Up for Sports,* was written for men and women who recognize the athlete in themselves. We often call these people "weekend athletes" because the time they have available for sports is limited. Author Ray Siegener has presented a logical approach to a safe, satisfying involvement with recreational sports. It is based on training methods that are—on the one hand—basic enough to be appropriate for the weekend athlete, yet are proven techniques endorsed by physical educators, trainers and athletes. The author challenges his reader with a proposition: "You don't play to get in shape," he says, "you get in shape to play." Whether your sport is tennis, golf, squash, skiing or hiking, you'll do it better, have more fun, less pain and enjoy it more if you incorporate a program of regular exercise into your life. All of our great amateur and professional athletes have accepted this necessity as a fact of life; the weekend athlete cannot afford to reject it.

One of the most exciting features of *Shape Up for Sports* is the author's utilization of some of America's leading athletes and sports figures to encourage the reader in his or her efforts toward personal fitness. Many of these stars have provided their own special warm-up and fitness tips and many of them appear in the illustrations as well. The exercises themselves are well presented and are compatible with the guidelines set down by the President's Council on Physical Fitness and Sports.

Recreational sports, by definition, should put relaxation, fun and pleasure into our lives. We all know that, for the untrained athlete, sports can do just the opposite. Physical activities that our bodies are not prepared for can cause muscle pulls, strains, tendonitis and even more tragic occurrences.

Most of us have to budget our time and allot the days and hours to a multitude of activities. This usually means weekend sports; but let's not accept the label "weekend athlete" for ourselves. If we're going to develop the *athlete* within each of us, it's a daily ritual, partly task... partly joy. We've got to train as athletes do. The daily jogging, calisthenics and stretching routines will not only help us to get there, but will be intensely rewarding in themselves.

James A. Lovell

Captain James A. Lovell, U.S.N. (Ret.) was commander of the Apollo 13 moon mission. He is the Special Consultant to the President on Physical Fitness and Sports.

SHAPE UP FOR SPORTS

CHAPTER 1

Shape Up for Sports— or Sports to Shape Up?

"I've got to do something about my gut," says the commuter in the bar car. "I think I'll take up tennis and get myself in shape." Similarly, the housewife or the businesswoman expresses concern at a tendency to "hippiness" and sees the tennis or racketball court as the answer.

What's wrong with that approach? Well, it probably won't work; and more important, it could be counterproductive. Most trainers and exercise physiologists agree that you don't play a sport to train, you train to play.

But Mr. Commuter isn't entirely off base. He has two ingredients in his equation that could add up to success if they are understood and positioned properly. First of all, he is aware that his physical condition leaves much to be desired—or better yet, to be attained. Second, he relates to a specific sport. Tennis must represent something to him. Perhaps he sees himself, lean and suntanned, sending an unreturnable backhand, just out of reach of the club's best player. A positive self-image. Fine. But if he's lost too much physically during his years of inactivity, his weekend tennis game is going to yield more pain than fitness, more frustration than great shots.

Let's look at the equation again: tennis = being in shape, and change it somewhat. Tennis and getting in shape = fun and feeling great and looking better. That one works. Sure, tennis will help us to get in shape if we appoint tennis as the reason to get in shape. The weekend tennis game or any other sport becomes part of the total picture which includes developing all the elements that the game requires: endurance, strength and flexibility.

1

What Do We Mean by Fitness?

Let's try some definitions on for size. The President's Council on Physical Fitness and Sports publishes a bulletin called the *Physical Fitness Research Digest.* Here's how the experts on the President's Council define physical fitness in that publication:

> Physical fitness is defined as the ability to carry out daily tasks with vigor and alertness, without undue fatigue, and with ample energy to enjoy leisure time pursuits and to meet unforeseen emergencies. Thus, physical fitness is the ability to last, to bear up, to withstand stress, and to persevere under difficult circumstances where an unfit person would quit. It is the opposite to becoming fatigued from ordinary efforts, to lacking energy to enter zestfully into life's activities, and to becoming exhausted from unexpected, demanding physical exertion.

The first reaction you might have to the above definition of fitness—before you apply it to sports or athletics—is that it sounds pretty darn good. How could anyone possibly want to feel any other way? As you'll see, most great athletes perceive fitness—and even the exercise it requires to get there—as a joyous thing. Paul Warfield, one of the most outstanding football players of the last decade, expressed his personal feelings on being fit: "Most people," said Paul, "and even some athletes in less physically demanding sports, go through life without knowing what it's like to be really physically fit. It is a rare joy, indeed, to experience a true feeling of fitness, regardless of what your sport is, and to find self-expression through that feeling. Many people accept and indulge in a moderate amount of exercise, but very few get even a glimpse of true fitness or find out what it's like to feel like a complete individual."

Paul Warfield has a perspective on fitness that will be with him throughout his lifetime, even when his football career is over and he is a weekend athlete like the rest of us. Sportscaster Frank Gifford, a one-time NFL All-Pro running back, now participates in sports for fun and for its fitness benefits. Frank told me: "As a former athlete I know the value of being physically fit. I try to stay active and involve myself in recreational activities which have fitness by-products. I play tennis several times a week and cycling provides the endurance-type activity that I need. Since I left professional football, my exercise isn't organized any longer, but it is regular."

Suzy Chaffee led our 1968 Olympic ski team to Grenoble. Since then she has been a World Champion free-style skier and, more recently, the hostess of her own TV series. Suzy admits, "Once I got to New York and the challenges of business, my fitness program was my salvation."

The athletes who have grown up as fit people and subsequently understood fitness as a vital component of their totality can sell fitness effectively. They know that being fit allows a person to stay involved with life at all levels.

There's No Age Limit on Fitness—or Sports

George Blanda, who recently retired from professional football, earned immense respect from fans and fellow athletes by playing that punishing sport until he was almost fifty years old. He is presently writing a book on fitness. George is living proof that staying fit keeps you in the game, so to speak. "I've always been an advocate of physical fitness," Blanda affirms. "I think my career will attest to that. I believe in not only a fitness program, but a recreation program for everyone. Fitness should be fun; that's why I say recreational program. You don't get into shape just to get through your everyday chores. You get into shape so that you can play tennis, so that you can bowl, so that you can play golf or go boating, or skating. You have to be in condition for these things, and if you're not in condition, you leave yourself open to injuries and other problems."

What is the relationship between age and fitness—or better yet, between fitness and aging? You may be surprised to learn that many ailments that were once attributed to aging are not due to chronological aging at all. They are the result of disuse.

In 1975 Dr. Lawrence E. Lamb, a prominent cardiologist and internist, author of many books on health and fitness and an adviser to the President's Council on Physical Fitness and Sports, delivered testimony to the Senate Subcommittee on Aging. Dr. Lamb pointed out that such maladies as heart disease, strokes, loss of physical ability, impotence and other signs of sexual decline, and loss of physical prowess are usually considered to be the consequences of aging. But all of these things are brought about prematurely by lack of physical activity. These disabilities and this kind of deterioration are "acquired changes" and not simply the result of passage of time. "These people," claims Dr. Lamb, "are not just getting older; they're sick." Dr. Lamb further testified that there is clear evidence of loss of muscle cells and decrease in size of muscles if they are not used, just as there is evidence that the amount of muscle mass can be increased with appropriate exercise. Disuse of the body not only affects skeletal muscles, but can affect the heart muscle, decreasing the heart's capacity. It can affect the lungs' capacity and almost every bodily system. Nature's rule is: if you don't use it, you lose it.

The good news is that much of the physical deterioration caused by lack of physical activity is reversible. With your physician's assistance and the right exercise program you can take up a sport and be physically ready for your sport. No matter what your chronological age is, you can slow the clock down with physical activity.

Elements of Fitness for Sport

A physical-fitness program for recreational sports should bring one to the level of physical readiness at which he or she can meet the physical demands of the sport without pain, injury or undue fatigue. In order to play at your sport, depending on what your sport is, you are going to have to develop the elements to appropriate levels. What are the elements of fitness that concern the weekend athlete? The *Physical Fitness Research Digest* outlines them in the following manner:

1. Muscular Strength. Muscular strength refers to the contraction power of muscles. How strong muscles are is usually measured with dynamometers or tensiometers, which record the amount of force particular muscle groups can apply in a single maximum effort.

    Man's existence and effectiveness depend upon his muscles. Movements of the body or any of its parts are impossible without action by muscles, attached to the skeleton. Muscles perform vital functions of the body as well. The heart is a muscle; death occurs instantly when it ceases to contract. Breathing, digestion and elimination are impossible without muscular contractions. And these vital functions are influenced by exercising the skeletal muscles: the heart beats faster, the blood circulates through the body at a greater rate, breathing becomes deep and rapid, and perspiration breaks out in the surface of the skin.
2. Muscular Endurance. Muscular endurance is the ability of the muscles to perform work. Two variations of muscular endurance are recognized: *isometric,* whereby a maximum static muscular contraction is held; and *isotonic,* whereby the muscles continue to raise and lower a (submaximal) load, as in weight training or performing pushups. Muscular endurance must assume some muscular strength. However, there are distinctions between the two. Muscle groups of the same strength may possess different degrees of endurance.
3. Circulatory-respiratory Endurance. Circulatory-respiratory endurance is characterized by moderate contractions of large muscle groups for relatively long periods of time, during which maximal adjustments of the circulatory-respiratory system are necessary, as in distance running or swimming.

In addition to the basic three above, other components of fitness include:

Muscular power: the ability to release maximum force in the shortest time. (Example: standing broad jump.)

Agility: speed in changing body positions or in changing directions. (Example: lateral movements on tennis court.)

Speed: rapidity with which successive movements of the same kind can be performed. (Example: fifty-yard dash.)

Flexibility: range of movements in a joint or a sequence of joints. (Examples: touch fingers to floor without bending knees, full body turn in golf swing.)

In order to present a practical program of exercises for the weekend athlete, I have reorganized the above into a three-part system by which it is possible to train effectively. Our conditioning program is comprised of the following:

1. *Warm-up and flexibility exercises.* These will provide a base from which you can exercise and engage in your sport with maximum range of motion and minimum risk of injury due to muscle pulls.
2. *Cardio-respiratory endurance.* Several methods of increasing endurance are suggested with emphasis on running. Your endurance program will allow you to engage in a weekly tennis game with energy and vigor and reduce risk of injury to the heart and its associated systems.
3. *Strength development.* Strength-development exercises are provided for both men and women. These routines will help the weekend athlete to play his sport with power and authority. It will help him or her to develop the physical strength to handle the stresses and strains of sport that can cause injury. Additionally, maintaining body strength and muscle tone is one of the ways we fend off the effects of aging.

If you follow the programs suggested in the following chapters, you will soon see dramatic effects reflected in your sports activities as well as in the way you feel. You will be developing cardio-respiratory fitness and you will be *stretching* and *strengthening* the muscle groups important to your athletic activities. In the chapters dealing with specific sports, special emphasis is placed on exercises that apply particularly to that sport.

Several years ago, the late Vince Lombardi, probably the most respected pro-football coach of all time, explained what fitness meant to his athletes and then related it to the layman. His words are certainly relevant to anyone involved in recreational sports. "A well-conditioned athlete," said Coach Lombardi, "is able to carry out his assignment properly, not only during the early part of the game, but right up until the final whistle. This is where he and his team really begin to enjoy an advantage: in the closing minutes of the game when they are still able to get off the ball crisply and block and tackle with authority and vigor. This is when your opponent knows he is beaten.

"A well-conditioned athlete has other things going for him. He *knows* he is ready to do whatever is necessary to beat his opponent. He knows he can wear his opponent down, if necessary. . . . I mention this only because all of us are required to function in some capacity. Whether you are a salesman, an office worker, an executive or a student, your daily routine makes certain demands of you . . . which you are ready to meet or not. It's that simple."

Begin with a Physical Examination

Anyone who has been inactive for any length of time and anyone over thirty years of age should begin their "shape-up" program with a visit to their physician. Your doctor will check your blood pressure, your pulse rate and may give you an EKG to check your heart functions. Show him this book and tell him how you plan to proceed with your fitness program, especially the endurance portion. Many physicians and exercise physiologists— Dr. Kenneth Cooper, the originator of "Aerobics," prominent among them—advise strongly that people in their thirties or forties or older be given a "stress" EKG before beginning a cardio-respiratory fitness program. A stress EKG measures and records the action of the heart under conditions that compare to those you experience when you exercise or play at your sport. If there is any malfunction of the heart and its associated systems, it should show up during a stress EKG. Discuss this with your physician. He will be able to arrange such an examination for you.

Once you have gotten the green light from your physician, you are ready to begin. Much of what you will be doing to "shape up for sports" will be work, but much of it will become a source of pleasure. Many people are finding a great deal of joy in developing and fine-tuning their physical capabilities. Dr. Sheehan said, "I returned to my body, and it changed my life." Chances are that, once you begin to see and feel results, you will become one of a growing number of people for whom fitness is an end—a joyful end—in itself.

CHAPTER 2

Prevention of Sports Injuries

To what degree are sports injuries preventable? Coaches, trainers, sports medical authorities and athletes themselves are continually addressing themselves to this question. Fortunately, as knowledge and techniques improve, the answer to that question becomes more encouraging. Many sports injuries can be prevented simply by applying the right off-season or pre-season conditioning program and by regular application of strengthening and stretching techniques to the muscle groups used in the various sports.

There are injuries that can occur as a consequence of outside forces (collisions, spills and contact-related accidents), and while conditioning may not seem to be a factor in such situations, the well-conditioned athlete is more likely to come out of an accident with fewer adverse effects. A limb with strong muscles and tendons and with good flexibility is more likely to be able to resist the stress, impact or torque which causes sprains, fractures and tears. Many people—even athletes and their trainers—are unaware that the bones themselves become stronger when the body is regularly subjected to resistance-type strengthening activities. While the Apollo Program was being conducted by the National Aeronautics and Space Administration, it was discovered that during the Apollo moon missions, measurable bone deterioration occurred in the bodies of the astronauts. Because of lengthy periods of relative physical inactivity, the bones tended to become weaker and porous. This condition is often observed in elderly people and has been thought to be a normal effect of the aging process. Here was stark evidence that another adverse physical condition formerly connected with aging was really attributable to inactivity. Fortunately for the astronauts and for millions of sedentary Americans, the process is reversible. Once the Apollo astronauts returned to their program of rigorous physical activity, their bone tissue became strong and solid again.

In this book we are concerned mainly with what we might think of as "self-inflicted" injuries—injuries that are caused by lack of conditioning or improper conditioning. The weekend athlete obviously is most susceptible to these kinds of injuries. Surprisingly for him or her, the answer to the injury problem will be found, to a great extent, in the chapters of this book dealing with flexibility, strength, and endurance. Right now we will explore the *why;* in the subsequent chapters you'll find the *how.*

Preventive Maintenance

Physical therapist Joseph Zohar has helped many of America's leading athletes to recover from sports-connected injuries. His theories on injury prevention are being adopted by trainers and team physicians in all phases of athletics. Here are Mr. Zohar's tips for what he calls "Trouble-free Sports Mileage":

> Athletes, like automobiles, require proper maintenance in order to perform continuously free of injury. Unfortunately, it appears that, at present, the average automobile driven in the United States receives better care than most athletes. . . . Programs designed to prevent athletic injuries are either nonexistent or inadequate.
>
> A preventive-maintenance for sports should include the following:
>
> 1. A pre-season preventive conditioning program consisting of stretching and progressive resistance exercise and special conditioning activities.
> 2. A pre-season examination by a qualified physician, including a complete range of motion test and an evaluation of the athlete's pre-season program.
> 3. A scaled-down preventive conditioning program during the season.
> 4. A full routine of warm-up exercises and activities prior to every practice and competitive event.

Mr. Zohar's approach was designed primarily for competitive athletes, but he is even more emphatic about the necessity for the weekend athlete to approach his sport in the same manner. He uses tennis and the high incidence of tennis-related injuries as a case in point.

> Common injuries, such as tennis elbow and shoulder tendonitis or bursitis, are usually caused by strains and stresses which exceed the tolerance of arm and shoulder muscles. The muscles are the primary force in the body's defense

mechanism against abnormal external forces which can cause injuries. Conditioning of muscles is, therefore, a key factor in preventing tennis injuries.

One may wonder, though, why even top professional and amateur players who are apparently in superior physical condition, nevertheless sustain injuries. The answer is quite simple. A chain is only as strong as its weakest link. All it takes is one muscle that is weak, tight, or lacks endurance, or an excessive imbalance in strength between opposing muscle groups, and an injury can occur. Unless all "weak links" are detected and corrected, a tennis player remains vulnerable to injury regardless of how superbly conditioned he appears to be.

The most effective way to prevent elbow and shoulder injuries is to increase the tolerance of *all* arm and shoulder muscles to levels far above and beyond the normal requirements of the game. To do so, each muscle group must be isolated and individually exercised until it reaches its highest desirable levels of strength, endurance, elasticity, capacity to relax and other desirable characteristics. This insures that no weakness, tightness or imbalance remain uncorrected. Similarly, many leg and back injuries can also be prevented by using a complete and balanced exercise program which combines progressive strengthening and stretching exercises.

Mr. Zohar's observations are valid for all athletes, especially weekend athletes, regardless of the nature of their sports. The stretching, strengthening and endurance exercises in the related chapters of this book will help you condition your body in the manner in which Joseph Zohar suggests and will minimize your injury risk.

Once we embark on a conditioning program that contains basic safeguards against sports injuries, we must examine the physical demands made by specific sports and the ways in which they relate to our physiology and our ability to deal with the stresses they will present to us. The legs and feet are particularly vulnerable to certain types of injury.

The Foot and the Leg

Foot and leg problems are unbelievably interrelated, so they should be presented in one dose to the weekend athlete.

Dr. George Sheehan, writer, marathon runner, cardiologist, the guru of distance runners in America and one of the pioneers in sports medicine—especially as it relates to the runner—has done some basic research on the leg and foot problems of runners and other athletes. This research, by the way, has largely been conducted firsthand by Dr. Sheehan at scores of marathon races. Dr. Sheehan has observed that many painful symptoms that runners and other athletes experience are traceable to the feet. "Many foot problems," Dr. Sheehan points out, "are due to a condition called 'Morton's foot,' which is characterized by a short first toe and a long second toe. It is basically a weak condition in the feet and causes all kinds of problems from stress fractures and heel spurs to Achilles tendonitis and knee disabilities." Surprisingly, the condition called Morton's foot is not rare; almost one-third of the population unknowingly has this foot weakness. Why don't all of these people experience pain or discomfort? Apparently, normal wear and tear on the foot—walking and occasional sports activities—do not exert the pressure and stress that cause the muscles and joints of the leg to break down. "Once you go into training," says Dr. Sheehan, "these things come out like images on a photographic plate." He recommends that anyone experiencing discomfort that may be traceable to Morton's foot visit a podiatrist.

The sports participant without congenital foot problems may still experience considerable discomfort and sometimes serious injury if his sport involves a great deal of running or if it requires sudden acceleration or deceleration or abrupt changes of direction.

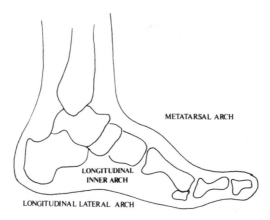

METATARSAL ARCH

LONGITUDINAL INNER ARCH

LONGITUDINAL LATERAL ARCH

THE ATHLETIC SHOE

There is probably nothing as important to your enjoyment of trouble-free and pain-free sports activity as a good, properly fitted athletic shoe. Here's what Dr. Sheehan advises regarding the relationship between shoes and foot-and-leg comfort for the athlete:*

> I hold it as an elemental rule that whatever a runner's disability is, it probably stems from his feet. There are, of course, exceptions. For instance, when there is acute trauma with pulls and sprains, and in the variety of sciatic pain syndromes. However, after these are eliminated, it is best to assume that any pain from the knee down comes from some difficulty with the feet.
>
> The foot is a marvelous mechanism which has 26 bones, and almost double that number of ligaments and muscles along with a few bursae that can bother the runner. In actual practice, however, the main difficulties originate in one of three arches.
>
> 1. *Longitudinal inner arch* along the inside of the foot extending from just in front of the heel to the base of the first long toe joint.
> 2. *Lateral longitudinal arch* in the same position on the outside of the foot.
> 3. *Metatarsal arch* across the ball of the foot.

*Reprinted from "Booklet of the Month," No. 1, *All About Distance Running Shoes,* 1971, pp. 38–39. By permission from *Runner's World* Magazine, P.O. Box 366, Mountain View, California 94040.

The longitudinal arch is bow-shaped and there is a sheet of tissue (the plantar fascia) that runs across the bottom of the foot, starting at the heel spur, like the string of the bow.

Part of the long arch is formed by the posterial tibial tendon that comes down the inside of the leg, hooks under the inside of the ankle bone and then proceeds across the bottom of the foot to the base of the fifth toe.

When the arch falls, this posterior tibial tendon is stretched. This produces pain which originally starts high on the inside of the calf, but over weeks or days as the arch falls, the pain gravitates down toward the ankle and eventually the pain gets into the arch proper and the plantar fascia is affected. At that point, it is almost impossible to run because of the pain.

At other times, the falling of the arch simply results in a turning in, or pronating, of the foot to a flat-foot position. This is an unnatural position for the rest of the leg and causes a shift of the mechanical stress, especially of the fibula and knee. In my book, this is the cause of chondromalacia of the knee and many stress fractures (although stress fractures may also be more related to an unstable foot).

Metatarsal arch problems are usually interpreted as bone bruises on the ball of the foot. Other difficulties associated with incorrect shoes are Achilles tendonitis from lack of heel lifts, especially in older runners, calluses from tight-fitting shoes, ingrown toenails from tight-fitting shoes and even loss of toenails from the same reason. The unstable foot can present a host of leg and foot pains, especially on the outside of the calf.

Blisters are a special problem, and I have handled that personally by taping the potentially affected areas with Zona tape (trainers' tape) prior to the event. Use of ladies' tennis socks or socks with reinforced bottoms has also been helpful. I stopped using vaseline when a new pair of shoes I bought came apart. Apparently, some shoes are glued together with a material which vaseline dissolves.

CONCLUSIONS:
1. Whenever disability occurs and whenever it manifests itself, the shoes should be considered the culprit unless proven otherwise.
2. Every runner is unique and may need help at one or all the arches of the foot.
3. When symptoms occur, the longitudinal arch support plus some additional heel lift would represent minimum care. These should be used in all shoes.
4. Expert care from a podiatrist with the use of an insert suitable for transfer from running shoes to daily shoes may be necessary, especially in severe cases involving chondromalacia and stress fractures.
5. Stretching the Achilles tendon and running on the outside of the foot will prevent many problems with the feet.

SELECTING THE SHOE

"The shoe, therefore, has to be a shoe that gives you support, and many of them don't," Dr. Sheehan states. "You need a shoe with a good heel because most people have a tight calf—especially women who have been wearing high heels. You need a heel that comes up about seven-eighths of an inch. You need a good shank so that it won't allow the foot to pronate too much. The shoe should have good shock absorption, but not too much stiffness. Some shoes have too much rubber under the ball of the foot, which can put strain on the Achilles. So there's a trade off between features in these shoes. But by and large, if you get a shoe that has good shock absorption, with a solid rubber shank, and a good-size heel with a fairly tight heel counter, you're well off.

"If you continue to experience discomfort in the knee or the muscle in the front of the shin, you can add a commercial arch support to your running shoes. The best one I know of is a Dr. Scholl #610. They are difficult to find, but they will help many foot and leg problems."

Recently, while I was traveling with Dr. Sheehan, we were approached by a young man with a rather sad story. The boy had been a World Class middle-distance runner until an injury forced him from amateur competitions. The nature of his injury points up the need for all sports participants—weekend athletes as well as professionals and amateurs—to give special attention to foot and leg maintenance. This individual, who was flirting with a World Record in his event, had never had a history of leg or foot disability. He was accustomed to running with a good, supportive running shoe with an adequate heel lift. One day, while vacationing in Florida, he decided that it would be fun to run barefoot on the beach. After running at a slow jog for ten miles or so, he began to experience severe pain in the Achilles tendon. The strain in the Achilles, caused by the runner's heels sinking into the sand whereas normally they had been elevated by a considerable heel lift, resulted in a tendonitis so severe that it meant the end of this young athlete's competitive career.

It may be necessary to spend close to thirty dollars for good running shoes (good tennis shoes are not nearly as expensive). But it would be difficult to put a dollar value on the avoidance of an excruciating case of Achilles tendonitis or "tennis toe."

Things to Watch Out For

HOT-WEATHER PROBLEMS

During most of our exercise and sports sessions, our bodies' temperature-regulating mechanisms are in control. They open the safety valves and allow us to perspire, which dissipates excess body heat. Our rate of perspiration adjusts to the degree of heat generated, and normally, breaking a sweat while exercising is not an unpleasurable feeling. Trouble begins when heat and humidity combine. When the air in which we are conducting our exercise or competition is saturated with moisture, it cannot effectively absorb the perspiration from our bodies. Without evaporation of perspiration, the body temperature begins to climb, triggering off increased perspiration. It is possible to lose two to three quarts of water in one hour of activity under these conditions. Some of the disabling effects of intense activity in hot, humid weather are:

1. Heat fatigue—a feeling of weakness brought about by the loss of water and salts.
2. Heat exhaustion—a condition caused by excessive loss of body salts and fluids, in which the athlete can become prostrated and unable to function.
3. Heat stroke—a failure of the body's cooling system. It is an *emergency situation* which can be fatal. It is recognized by hot, dry skin and loss of consciousness.

The most effective way to ward off adverse physical reactions to hot weather is to replace body fluids and salts constantly. One of the unfortunate myths among athletes has been that you should never drink fluids while involved in a contest or a heavy workout. This old-wives' tale is probably traceable to the negative effect of drinking *too much* ice-cold water or other beverage during periods of intense activity. Of course, that kind of thing is not recommended, but it is essential to replace the amount of body fluids that are being lost through perspiration.

You can replace the other elements lost with body fluids by drinking lightly salted water, fruit juice or any of the "gatorade" type drinks prepared for athletes. Beware of salt tablets—they can cause intestinal and other problems.

Approach hot-weather activities and training with common sense and patience, and before long, your body will have adjusted to its environment.

Cold-Weather Problems

The effects of cold weather can be just as serious as those brought about by excess heat. Joggers, skiers and skaters are most susceptible to cold-weather difficulties. One of the reasons that snow shoveling claims so many coronary victims each winter is that extreme cold places extra stress on the heart. Blood vessels supplying the heart muscle are constricted and blood is shunted to other parts of the body. So whether you are shoveling snow, jogging or skiing cross-country, don't push yourself when the weather is bitterly cold.

Frost bite is another hazard to watch out for in cold weather. When you are jogging on a cold day, you force air into and out of your lungs very rapidly. The air you breathe doesn't have a chance to become warmed. It is possible to experience frost bite of throat and lung tissue if the temperature is well below freezing.

The extreme example of adverse effect from cold temperatures is hypothermia, which means that the body's heat-producing system is not keeping up with heat losses. It is analogous to heat stroke in that it is an emergency situation and can be fatal. Inadequate clothing and inexperience with extreme cold usually are the causes of hypothermia.

SHIN SPLINTS

Since many readers are joggers or runners, and since the endurance-development program recommended in this book is a walking-jogging-running program, a word about shin splints is in order. The term "shin splints" covers a multitude of painful situations. Symptomatically, they all feel the same: soreness in the lower portion of the shin bone. The AMA's *Standard Nomenclature of Athletic Injuries* defines shin splints as an inflammation of the muscles leading from the shin (tibia) to the foot, which results from unaccustomed repetitive activity (such as running on hard surfaces). Shin splints are a common ailment and most joggers and runners experience them at one time or another. Best remedies are as follows:

1. Rest for a day or two, or until the pain is no longer troublesome.
2. Strengthen shin muscles. (See section titled "Special Tips for Runners" in the "Special Tips" chapter.
3. Increase flexibility of antagonist (calf muscles). (See "Special Tips for Runners.")
4. Refer to Dr. Sheehan's comments on athletic shoes in this chapter.
5. Give attention to footstrike (roll from heel to toe) to avoid pounding. You may have to shorten your stride to do this.

BLISTERS

Normally, a blister would be considered a minor problem. For the weekend athlete it's not minor. Why? Because so many sports and fitness programs have been totally destroyed by pain. When a scholastic or professional athlete has trouble with blisters, he gets treatment and then accepts the discomfort as part of the job. When a newcomer to athletics or fitness activities experiences pain, he or she is likely to say, "This isn't for me!" A blister can start out as a small pain and grow into such a nuisance that it literally knocks the pins out from under your conditioning or sports program.

Blisters can often be avoided. If they occur, they should be treated immediately. The avoidance of blisters—as with many other sports ailments—begins with the shoes. Make sure that you give attention to the following:

1. Make sure shoes are fitted properly. This is elementary. Shoes should not slip or pinch. The break in the sole should coincide with the bend in your foot—right under the ball.
2. Break new shoes in slowly. Have an extra pair.
3. If the feet are tender, wear two pairs of socks. A pair of cotton socks next to the skin with a pair of wool socks over the cotton works quite well.
4. Examine the feet after you run, ski, play tennis and so on and look for any red areas or

sore spots. If you find such areas, try to locate the cause of the irritation. Perhaps a change of shoes would help.

If blisters do form, the best way to deal with them is to have medical advice. Your physician can treat blisters without risk of infection. He should be able to advise you as to whether a foot powder or a lubricant would help to avoid reoccurrence.

ALCOHOL—IS IT A PROBLEM?

Recent studies at the University of California revealed that the ingestion of alcohol had radical effects on the efficiency of the heart action. Two ounces of alcohol increased the resting heart rate and the amount of oxygen consumed by the heart muscle with the body at rest. This is the kind of information we may or may not welcome, but in any case, we've got a way to put it to the test.

The Vanderbilt YMCA (New York City) *Fitness Newsletter* suggests the following: "Take your resting heart rate, then have a cocktail. Wait 15 to 20 minutes and check your pulse rate again. The increased rate is an indication of the increased work."

Weekend athletes may want to reposition the use of alcohol as they set up training schedules and competitive activities.

*Danger Signs and What to Do**

1. Abnormal heart function—fluttery, irregular pulse.
    —fluttery feeling in chest or throat.
    —rapid heartbeat.
    —sudden, very slow heartbeat, either immediately after exercises or later.

2. Chest pain
    —any pain or unusual pressure in the chest.
    —pain or pressure in the arm or throat after exercise.

3. Dizziness
    —any feeling of light-headedness.
    —confusion or incoordination.
    —cold sweat.
    —pallor, blueness or loss of consciousness.

If any of the above occur, stop exercise immediately and call physician.

*Adapted from "Exercise Your Way to Fitness and Heart Health" by Lenore Zohman, M.D., 1974.

4. Persistent rapid pulse —retention of rapid heart rate 5–10 minutes after exercise is finished.

Remedy: Exercise is too intense. Increase rate of intensity more slowly. Consult physician if problem persists.

Summary of Pointers for Safe and Injury-Free Sports Training

Recently the President's Council on Physical Fitness and Sports published a set of guidelines for training and exercise developed by Thomas K. Cureton, Ph.D. Dr. Cureton is a member of the Council's clinic staff and has been described as an "evangelist for physical fitness." Here is Dr. Cureton's list of rules for exercise, which have gotten thousands of people safely to their fitness goals.

1. Warm-up Rule: take it easy, 15 to 20 minutes, walk before you run, at least do some preliminary bending, stretching, running in place. Warm-up is protective against injuries and the sudden development of an oxygen deficiency.
2. Regulation of Dosage: Build up the intensity of the work gradually; then push up to a peak of effort; then taper off. Several ways to regulate the work are:

   - Walk a lap (block) and jog a block; repeat several times.
   - Then walk several blocks (laps).
   - Walk a lap (block) and jog 2; walk a block and jog 3; walk a block and jog 4; etc. Then, walk several laps.
   - Take a long jog, continuous running.
   - Do repetitious fast runs with walks between.
   - Cross-country run, walk, jog.

3. Rule for Progressively More Work: Improvement depends upon a gradual increase in the total amount of work done. The progression is equivalent to 100, 300, 500 calories of heat, corresponding to 30 minutes, 45 minutes, an hour of work with gradual increase in intensity.
4. Recuperation Rule: Keep moving, don't sit down; go from the gym to the showers (hot, then cold) and swim a few minutes, if possible. Breathe as deeply as possible and force the breath out explosively. Stretch any muscles which have been worked out. Avoid smoking, which constricts lung capillaries.
5. Work Various Parts: Neck, shoulders, chest, upper back, waist, lower back, abdomen, legs and feet. In addition, there should be some running (perhaps in

place) or rowing, skating, swimming, cycling, skiing—some continuous rhythmical work for endurance, forcing the circulation and respiration.

6. Rule for Heart Protection: Warm up gradually before exposure to hard work, or extreme cold or extreme heat; avoid severe tensions longer than a few seconds at a time; and try to get enough ventilation for the work being done. Medical exam is recommended.

7. Rule for Deep Breathing: Time breathing with each exercise so as to get as full and deep ventilation as possible. This wards off fatigue.

8. Use of Fuel: To use up fuel (food), it is a matter of 1 to 15 calories burned per minute, depending upon the intensity of the exercise. The length of time one exercises at a given rate determines how much fuel is used. To burn one pound of fat requires 4,320 to 4,380 calories, according to the respiratory efficiency. To burn fat reserves takes time. There is no shortcut.

9. Posture Rule: Posture should be relaxed enough to permit good circulation. Strength is needed for the posture-maintaining muscles to resist gravity for any length of time. Posture muscles should be trained: neck, shoulders, abdomen, seat, thighs, and supinators of the feet.

10. Flexibility Rule: Daily stretching is needed. Any muscle which is held motionless or tensed for very long will become stiff. Flexibility may diminish with age, but it may be maintained by daily stretching all joints. It is better to warm-up and then stretch. Stretching in a warm room or under the water is good.

11. Emotional Rule: Avoid severe emotions, if possible, but, if they are brewing, take a walk or leave the scene. Strong emotions are doubly dangerous in unfit people (increased blood pressures because of mental state). Keep fit to stand your emotions—it helps.

12. Strength Rule: Strength is developed by working against high resistance, lifting loads, pushing and pulling (as with barbells, medicine balls, pulleys, resistance machines and partner exercises). The muscles must be used *hard*. Casual housework or easy running is not sufficient.

13. Glandular-Fitness Rule: Hard exercise stirs up the sympathetic nervous system and also affects the glandular functions. Adrenal function is highly related to endurance. Cold baths, endurance work and sufficient iodine intake are important; and use develops function.

14. Maximum-Respiration Rule: In hard work, maximum breathing is needed to last and to be as protected as possible. Force the breathing in every hard exercise, and avoid holding the breath during a strength effort.

15. Maximum-Circulation Rule: Circulation is usually better in the lying rather than the sitting or standing position. It is better in a cool environment than a hot environment. Rhythmic movement is the greatest boost to circulation, but tense (static) efforts may block the circulation more or less. Forced breathing helps the circulation along with walking, running, swimming, skating, skiing, dancing, rowing and rhythmic calisthenics.

16. Use Your Own: Your own muscles must do the work for best results; don't depend upon passive massage, manipulation, heat or vibration devices.

17. Time of Workout: Best for most people is about 3–4 hours after meals; but people who sit nearly all day need to get up and move about at least every hour, and if possible, every few minutes. Many work before breakfast, or at 12 to 1 P.M.; and many work at night 9 to 10 P.M. One can adapt to any reasonable schedule. Avoid hard work right after meals.
18. Take Cool Baths: Normally baths should be hot (short), then cool (long) as cool baths are recuperative, help the circulation and stir up the metabolism more than hot baths; but a hot bath is all right just before bed.
19. Fortify the Diet: The harder and harder the work, the more fortification of the diet is needed with vitamin B-complex, C and such boosters as wheat germ and wheat-germ oil.
20. Include Protective Foods: Red, green, yellow vegetables; milk; lean meat.

First-Aid Chart for Athletic Injuries

The first-aid tips suggested below were developed by the AMA Committee on the Medical Aspects of Sports in cooperation with the National Athletic Trainers Association and the National Federation of State High School Athletic Associations.

BONES AND JOINTS

Fracture: never move athlete, if fracture of back, neck or skull is suspected. Obtain medical care at once.

Neck: Maintain the neck in the plain of the body, neither flexing nor hyper-extending to correct.

Dislocation: Support joint. Apply ice bag or cold cloths to reduce swelling, and refer to physician.

Bone bruise: Apply ice bag or cold cloths and protect from further injury. If severe, refer to physician.

Broken nose: Apply cold cloths and refer to physician.

CARDIAC ARREST

Mouth-to-mouth resuscitation is mandatory when definite cardiac arrest can be determined. Emergency aid should be summoned at the first sign of cardiac arrest.

Mouth-to-mouth resuscitation:

The procedure is as follows:
1. Place the victim face up.
2. Tilt head back.
3. Take a deep breath and pinch victim's nose.
4. Blow in until chest rises.
5. Remove your mouth and let victim exhale.
6. When victim has exhaled, replace your mouth on his, pinch his nose and repeat.
7. Repeat 15 times per minute.

IMPACT BLOWS

Head: If any period of dizziness, headache, uncoordination or unconsciousness occurs, disallow any further activity and obtain medical care at once. Keep the athlete lying down; if unconscious, give nothing by mouth. If there is inequality of the pupils or drift of the outstretched hand with the eyes closed, then this is an emergency situation.

Teeth: Save teeth if completely removed from socket. If loosened, do not disturb; cover with sterile gauze and refer to a dentist at once.

Celiac plexus: Rest athlete on back and moisten face with cool water. Loosen clothing around waist and chest. Do nothing else except obtain medical care if needed.

Testicle: Rest athlete on back and apply ice bag or cold cloths. Obtain medical care, if pain persists.

Eye: If vision is impaired, refer to physician at once. With soft tissue injury, apply ice bag or cold cloths to reduce swelling.

HEAT ILLNESSES

Heat stroke: Collapse WITH DRY WARM SKIN indicates sweating-mechanism failure and rising body temperature. THIS IS AN EMERGENCY; DELAY COULD BE FATAL. Immediately cool athlete by the most expedient means (immersion in cool water is best method). Obtain medical care at once.

Heat exhaustion: Weakness WITH PROFUSE SWEATING indicates state of shock due to depletion of salt and water. Place in shade with head level or lower than body. Give sips of dilute salt water, if conscious. Obtain medical care at once.

Sunburn: If severe, apply sterile gauze dressing; refer to physician.

Muscles and Ligaments

Bruise: Apply ice bag or cold cloths, and rest injured muscle. Protect from further aggravation. If severe, refer to physician.

Cramp: Have opposite muscles contracted forcefully, using firm hand pressure on cramped muscle. If during hot day, give sips of dilute salt water. If recurring, refer to physician.

Strain and sprain: Elevate injured part and apply ice bag or cold cloths. Apply pressure bandage to reduce swelling. Avoid weight bearing and obtain medical care.

Open Wounds

Heavy Bleeding: Apply sterile pressure bandage using hand pressure, if necessary. Refer to physician at once.

Cut and abrasion: Hold briefly under cold water, then cleanse with mild soap and water. Apply sterile pad firmly until bleeding stops, then protect with more loosely applied sterile bandage. If extensive, refer to physician.

Puncture wound: Handle same as cuts, and refer to physician.

Nosebleed: Keep athlete sitting or standing; cover nose with cold cloths. If bleeding is heavy, pinch nose and place small cotton pack in nostrils. If bleeding continues, refer to physician.

Other Concerns

Blisters: Keep clean with mild soap and water and protect from aggravation. If already broken, trim ragged edges with sterilized equipment. If extensive or infected, refer to physician.

Foreign body in eye: Do not rub. Gently touch particle with point of clean, moist cloth and wash with cold water. If unsuccessful or if pain persists, refer to physician.

What About Nutrition and the Pre-Game Meal?

The weekend athlete's main concern with diet and nutrition should be: what kind of diet is going to make me healthy? The first thing you will find out about diet, once you begin a serious exercise program, is that you are going to care a lot more about what you eat. If you spend a half-hour each morning running and another half-hour at your flexibility and strength-development programs, you are going to develop an increased awareness of your body—in ways that you probably can't imagine. You are not going to want to put foods into your body that are going to undermine and sabotage all the positive things you are doing. When asked about his training diet, the great miler Marty Liquori said, "I know what I shouldn't eat." That's really where it's at. We all know what we shouldn't eat. We all know about the so-called "balanced diet," and we also know that it is becoming more and more difficult—in this age of synthetic and highly processed foods—to know if we are achieving it or not.

The weekend athlete has heard a lot about various kinds of diets for athletes. There are high-fat, high-protein and high-carbohydrate diets and low versions of all of these. What the weekend athlete should know is that his weekly tennis game or golf match isn't going to be drastically affected by his pre-game meal. If you are going to run a six-mile road race or engage in any kind of "long-duration" event, that is something else altogether. Most coaches and trainers of distance runners and swimmers are recommending that their athletes eat foods high in fats and proteins for the first four days of the week before a race and then switch to a diet high in carbohydrates for the last three days. This technique is called "carbohydrate loading" and seems to be attaining some acceptance as a method of achieving "long-duration" performance.

Recreational athletes who are into serious running, swimming, squash or tennis will be interested in Dr. Sheehan's thoughts on the pre-game meal: "Your approach to the pre-game meal should be to take something that you know agrees with you. The second thing is that you want to compete on an empty stomach. It takes about three or four hours for the stomach to empty, and if you're nervous, it might take longer. So, for your pre-game meal, take something that agrees with you, with emphasis on carbohydrates rather than fats or proteins, about four hours before. Now, this does not include fluids. Fluids are essential and can be taken while you are competing, and in hot weather you should begin your fluid intake about ten minutes before you begin. On a hot humid day try about ten ounces of water or a half-strength ade or orange juice. Then take ten ounces more about every twenty minutes."

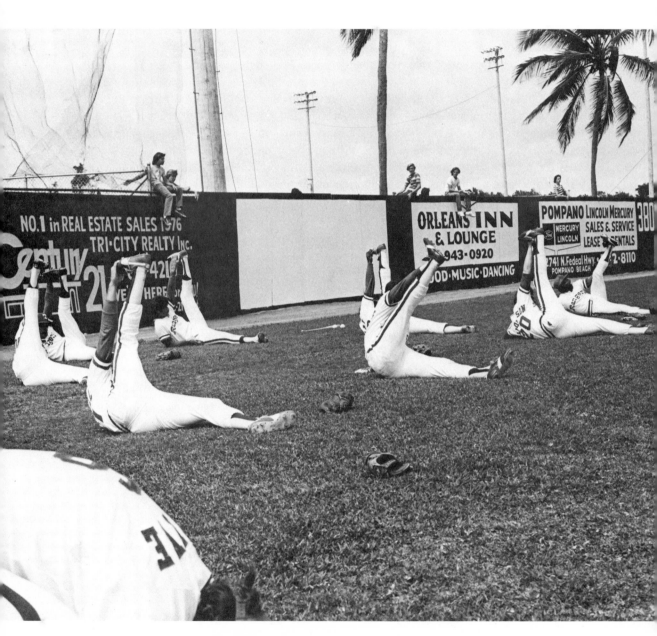

Texas Rangers consider flexibility routine a vital part of daily workout.

CHAPTER 3

Warm-up and Flexibility Exercises

The main thing for the weekend athlete is loosening up the body. Nowadays, even professionals who are very active are more aware of this than in the past. Before a game you'll see the guys limbering up and doing lots of stretching exercises. There are certain types of injuries that occur when you don't stretch . . . groin injuries, calf injuries and many other kinds of muscle pulls.

For example, I haven't had a muscle pull in the last four years and that's primarily due to the fact that before each game I do my flexibility and stretching exercises. I always stretch my Achilles tendon, an exercise which is very important as you grow older. You find a lot of weekend athletes experiencing torn Achilles tendons because they haven't been exercising that part of their bodies. They go out on the tennis or squash court; they reach for the low shot and they have a problem.

Earl Monroe, New York Knicks

Athletes and coaches have always known about the need for warm-up exercises. Indeed, Myron's Discus Thrower probably checked out the fairways at a slow jog before sending his stone quoit ranging through the rarified air of Olympia. Warm-ups are now part of the scientific method as applied to modern athletics. We know why warm-ups are important. They do what athletes have always known that they did: they elevate the body temperature, they increase respiration and get all systems ready to go.

Cool, unprepared muscles and an unsuspecting circulatory-respiratory system should never be subjected to the sudden demands of an active sport or the shock of intense endurance or strength exercises. Warm-up routines should be part of each conditioning session; they should also precede every round of golf and each session on the tennis courts or the ski slopes. No matter what your sport is, you can't afford to neglect the warm-up. Not only do you run the risk of pulled muscles and other injuries, you just won't function well until you get your body up to speed.

Introduction to Flexibility

In a sense, flexibility routines are an extension of the warm-up concept. In recent years, they have become a vital part of the training process. Athletes, trainers and coaches, as well as physicians and physical therapists engaged in sports medicine, have discovered a significant fact concerning muscular conditioning. In simple terms, what happens is that as a muscle is strengthened through incorrect training or use in sports activities, it may become shorter and less resilient. To compound the problem, the muscle's opposite number (muscle pairs usually function as flexors and extensors around a joint) often becomes relatively weaker because it is trained less intensely. Now we have a situation in which an injury is likely, if not inevitable: an antagonistic muscle pair (flexor and extensor), one of which is strong but with limited flexibility, the other being weak and poorly trained. It's an accident waiting to happen. What can be done about this? Two things. The body's weak muscles can be strengthened by means of calisthenics and weight-training techniques, as outlined in the "Strength Development" chapter in this book. Then, by regularly doing a series of stretching and flexibility exercises such as the routines that follow, muscles in the entire body will become longer and more resilient and less likely to react adversely to the stresses that your sport will place on them.

If the warm-up is intended to loosen up the athlete so as to prepare him for his workout or sports activity, the flexibility exercises are intended to have a longer-range effect. They will stretch the muscles so that pulling and tearing is less likely; they will facilitate full range of movement so that the athlete becomes more dexterous and more proficient at his or her sport.

Begin Your Program with Flexibility

Many people who have been turned on to sports activities and/or fitness for its own sake end up being casualties before they ever really get started. We live in an age of instant gratification—in a time when rapid achievement of goals is considered meritorious. Fitness doesn't work that way. Athletics is an uncompromising area of life. You can't fake it. The pole-vaulter either can get over the bar or he can't.

If a person wants to reach physical goals, he or she must put in the time. It's surprising how pleasant it is to see and feel your body improving—becoming stronger, leaner and looser. Try to hurry that process and you pay a price. The price is pain—and failure.

If you are considering a total-fitness program—one including endurance and strength development as well as improvement in flexibility and agility—you may be well advised to begin right here, in this chapter. The number of well-intentioned people who have embarked on running and weight-training programs only to be stymied by pain, by stiffness, strains, back problems and tendonitis, are legion.

Try this. Begin your fitness program with the warm-up and stretching exercises in this chapter. Do them for two weeks. You don't have to be able to do all of them. After two weeks you will be amazed at how much looser you feel and how your body seems to be much more under control. Then begin the other elements of your fitness program. Your running program and strength-development activities should be pleasant and fun to do. They should satisfy psychological as well as physical needs. And they will, if you're not distracted or discouraged by pain.

Recommended Warm-ups and Flexibility Exercises for Men and Women

This flexibility program is suitable for men and women. The exercises are demonstrated on these pages by former Olympic and World Champion free-style skier, Suzy Chaffee, and by Tug McGraw, Philadelphia Phillies relief pitcher. They are the basic exercises now used by National Football League teams, Major League baseball teams and most world-class athletes in tennis, soccer, track and field, basketball, hockey and skiing. Before you begin, here are some important facts that you should learn and remember about flexibility:

1. Stretching the muscles is a slow process. Don't try to do any exercise that appears to be too difficult. Work up to the hard ones.
2. Don't "bounce" on a muscle as you try to stretch it. Your sensation should be that of a slight, steady pulling action.
3. Do each exercise two or three times, unless otherwise instructed.
4. Try to stretch a little bit further on each successive session, until obvious limits are reached. As you progress, you'll reach positions that you would never have believed possible.
5. You can do these exercises daily and they feel so good you probably will; but try to do them at least three times a week.
6. Begin your flexibility routine with a warm-up. The first four exercises are part of the warm-up and should be included in all of your "on-court" and "off-court" warm-ups.

WARM-UP SESSION

Jog in place for two minutes or do an easy jog around the track for 200 yards. This will stimulate circulation and respiration.

- Stand with arms outstretched and flex fingers.
- Flex and rotate wrists.
- Make small circles with extended arms. Allow to grow into giant circles.

Proceed with the following exercises:

1. Side Bends

Starting position: Stand erect with hands at sides, feet spread to shoulder width.
Action:
(1) Bend the trunk to the right until resistance is felt.
(2) Return to upright position.
(3) Bend the trunk to the left.
Suggested repetitions: Begin with 10, work up to 20-30.

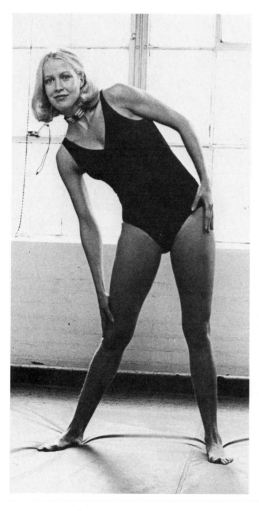 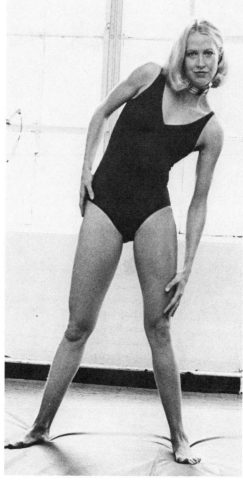

2. Hip Thrusts

Starting position: Stand erect with hands at sides, feet spread comfortably apart.
Action:
(1) Slowly bend the body back, while thrusting pelvis forward and raising hands high over the head. Exhale during this action. Hold for several counts.
(2) Return to starting position. Inhale and rest for 3–5 counts.
Suggested repetitions: 10.
Note: This exercise can be done with hands on hips throughout.

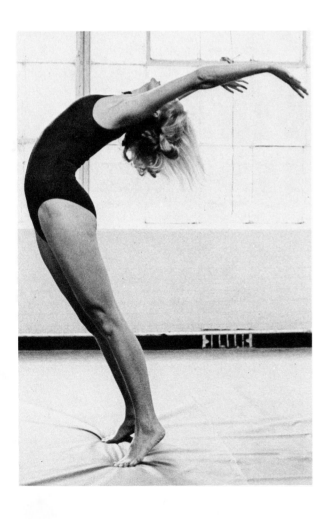
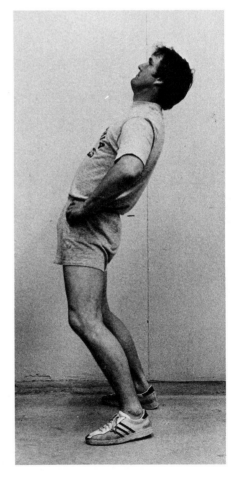

3. Flexed-Leg Back Stretch

Starting position: Stand erect with arms at sides.
Action:
(1) Slowly bend over and touch your fingertips to the floor, while exhaling. Your knees should be bent slightly. You'll feel a comfortable stretching effect in the lower back and back of legs. Hold for 15–20 counts.
(2) Return to starting position while inhaling. Rest for 5–10 counts and then repeat.
Suggested repetitions: 2–3.

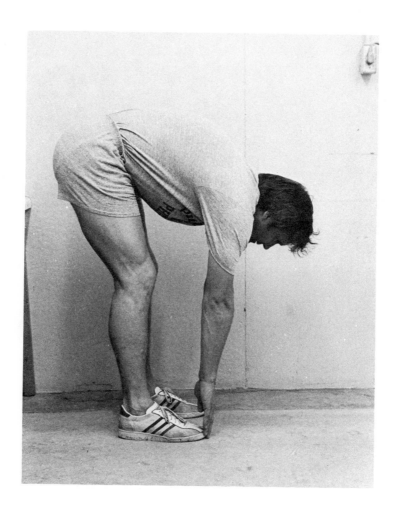

4. Trunk Twister

Starting position: Stand erect with feet at shoulder width. Extend arms straight out from your sides.

Action:

(1) Slowly turn the upper part of the body to the right as far as you can, without straining. Keep feet stationary.

(2) Slowly turn the upper body to the left, again without straining.

Suggested repetitions: 10–15 each side.

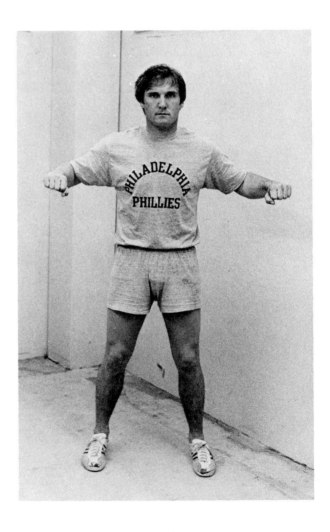

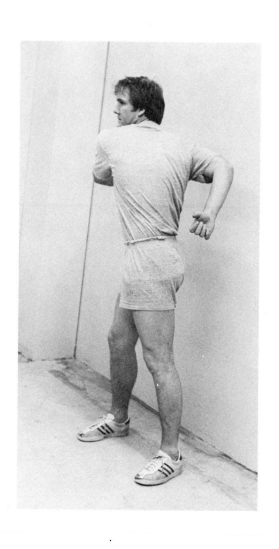
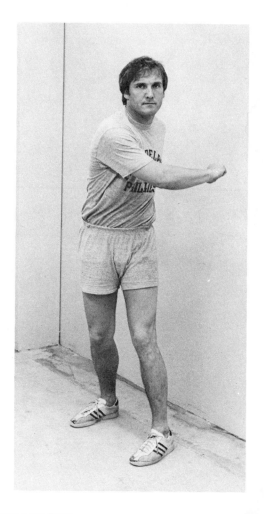

5. Alternate Knee Pull

Starting position: Lie on back, legs extended, hands at side.
Action:
(1) Pull one leg to chest, grasp leg with both arms and hold for a 5 count.
(2) Repeat with other leg.
Suggested repetitions: 7–10 with each leg.

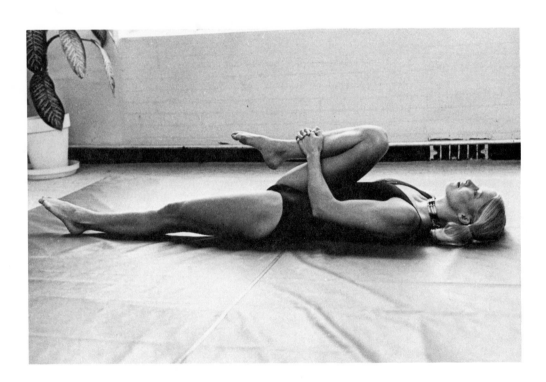

6. Double Knee Pull

Starting position: Lie on back, legs extended, hands at sides.
Action:
Pull both legs to chest, lock arms around legs, pulling buttocks slightly off the floor.
Hold for 20–40 counts.
Suggested repetitions: 7–10 times.

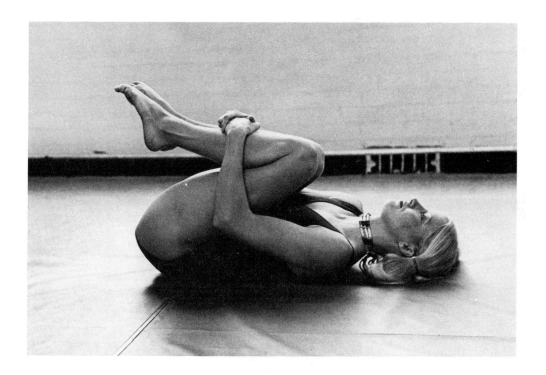

7. Achilles Stretch

Starting position: Stand at arms length from wall, with both palms pressed against wall.

Action:

(1) Move one leg forward ½ step, move opposite leg back ½ step.
(2) With heel of rear leg held to the floor, lean toward wall, stretching calf muscle and Achilles tendon.
(3) Hold for 5–10 counts.
(4) Reverse leg position and repeat.

Suggested repetitions: 3–6 each leg.

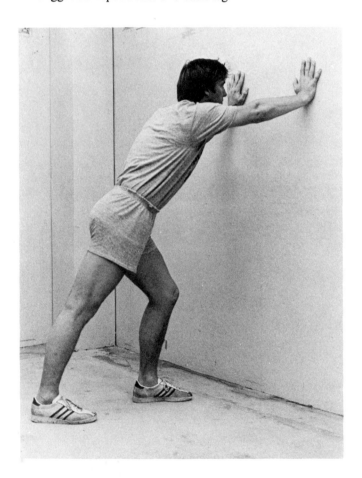

8. Prone Back Arch

Starting position: Lie flat on the floor, face down with legs and feet extended.
Action:
(1) While exhaling, straighten arms and arch the back until elbows are straight.
(2) Tip head back as far as possible, without straining neck muscles.
(3) Hold for 5–10 counts.
(4) Inhale as you return to starting position.
Suggested repetitions: 4–6.

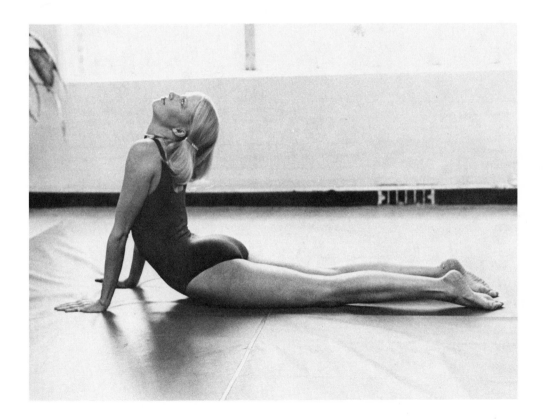

9. Hip Rotators

Starting position: Sit on floor with upper body weight supported by arms and hands, legs extended.

Action:

(1) Bring knees close to body until feet almost contact buttocks.

(2) Rotate legs and hip to the right, bringing right knee as close to the floor as possible.

(3) Rotate legs and hip to the left so that left knee comes as close to the floor as possible.

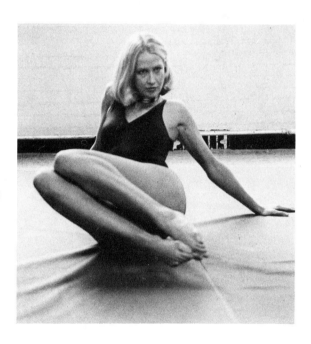
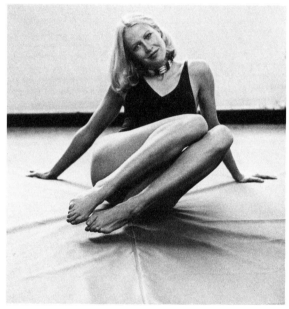

10. Seated Pike Stretch

Starting position: Sit on floor with legs extended and feet together.
Action:
(1) While exhaling, lean forward slowly, sliding hands down legs toward the ankles.
(2) Try to touch the chin to knees, while keeping the legs as straight as possible.
(3) Without "bouncing," hold 5–10 counts.
(4) Inhale while returning to starting position.
Suggested repetitions: 4–6.

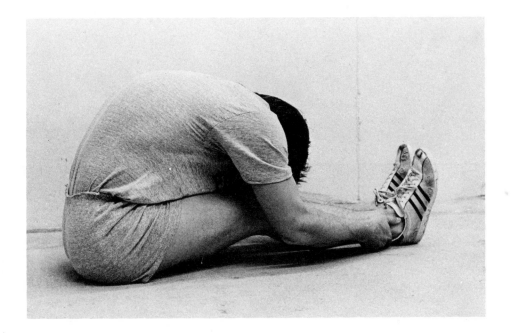

11. Head-to-Floor Stretch

Starting position: Sit on floor with legs spread wide apart.
Action:
(1) While exhaling, bend forward, sliding hands down ankles.
(2) Try to touch forehead to floor, while keeping legs as straight as possible.
(3) Hold position for 5–10 counts.
(4) Inhale deep, while returning to starting position.
Suggested repetitions: 4–6.
Note: Don't be discouraged if you cannot get your forehead down to the floor. Lower it as far as possible, without straining. As your flexibility increases, you'll come closer to the goal.

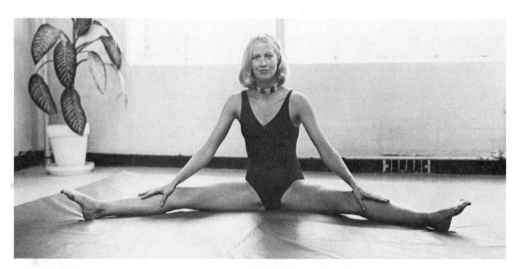

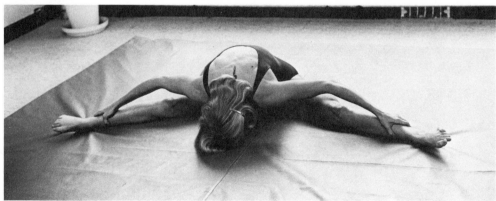

12. Alternate Hamstring Stretch

Starting position: Sit on floor as for previous exercise.
Action:
(1) While exhaling, bend forward over right leg, sliding hands down to right ankle.
(2) Touch chin to right knee, keeping right leg as straight as possible.
(3) Without "bouncing," hold for 10–15 counts.
(4) Inhale while returning to starting position.
(5) Repeat with left leg.

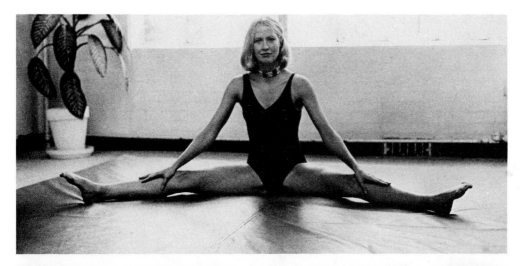

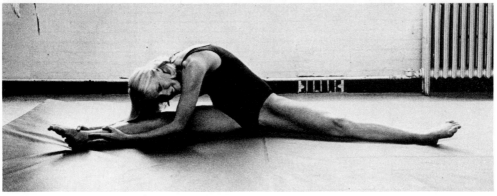

13. Hurdler's Stretch

Starting position: Sit on the floor, as illustrated, with right leg extended forward and left bent to the side with foot behind buttock.

Action:

(1) While exhaling, bend forward over right leg, sliding both hands down leg to right ankle.
(2) Touch chin to right knee, keeping knee as straight as possible.
(3) Hold for 5–10 counts.
(4) While inhaling, return to starting position.
(5) Repeat, with leg positions reversed.

Suggested repetitions: 3–5 in each position.

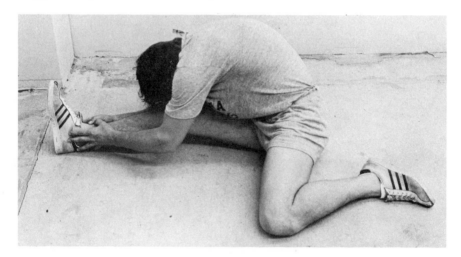

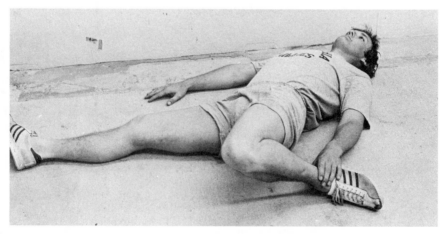

14. Hand-to-Foot Stretch and Balance

Starting position: Stand erect with left foot held in left hand, right arm extended for balance or used for support against a wall or chair.

Action:

(1) Bend forward as far as possible, while maintaining balance. Try to bring foot up to shoulder height.

(2) Return to starting position.

(3) Repeat, while holding right foot.

Suggested repetitions: 2–3 with each leg.

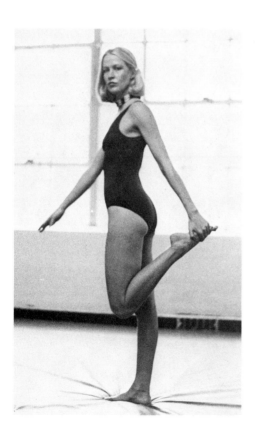
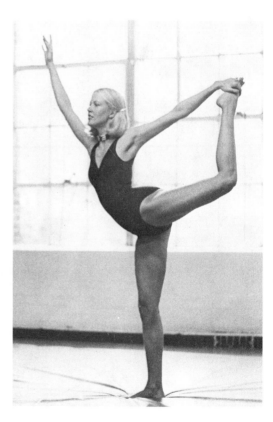

15. Side Leg Stretch

Starting position: Stand erect with feet spread wider than shoulder width, right arm extended out to the side, left arm extended straight ahead.
Action:
(1) Stretch to left, bending left leg and keeping right leg extended until moderate pulling is felt inside thigh and groin area.
(2) Return to starting position.
(3) Repeat, with arm and leg positions reversed.
Suggested repetitions: 10–15 each side.
Note: Suzy demonstrates this exercise with arms extended, as shown; many athletes prefer to perform this drill with hands on hips.

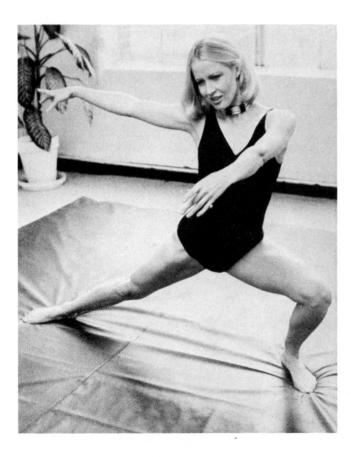

16. Backover

Starting position: Lie on floor, with arms extended over head.
Action:
(1) While exhaling, bring legs over head and as close as possible to the floor.
(2) Hold for 5 counts.
(3) While inhaling, return to starting position.
Suggested repetitions: 2–3.

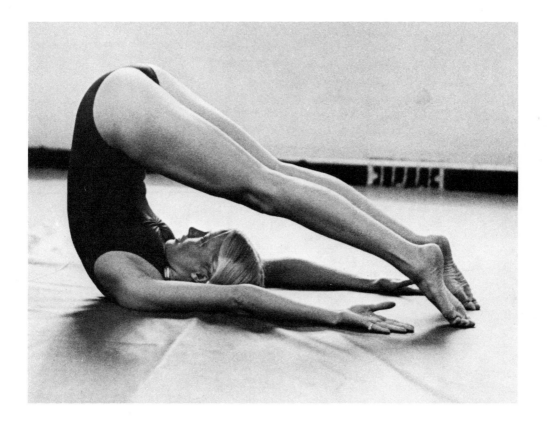

17. Back Arch

Starting position: Lie on floor with legs positioned as illustrated and palms of hands near shoulders.
Action:
(1) Press body up into an arch so that arms and legs are extended.
(2) Hold for 5 counts.
(3) Return to starting position.
Suggested repetitions: 2–3.

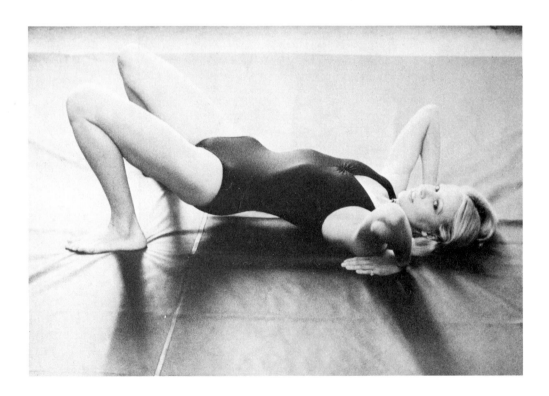

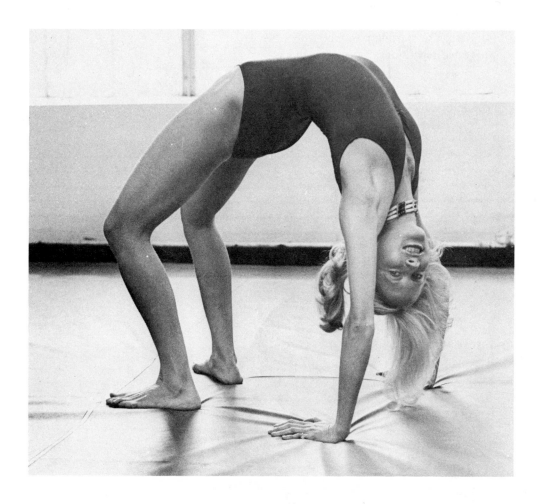

18. Upright Leg Stretch

Starting position: Stand erect with right leg extended and right foot supported by the back of a chair or other object of suitable height.
Action:
(1) Slide hands down leg to right ankle.
(2) Bend forward, bring head as close to right knee as possible.
(3) Hold for 10–15 counts.
(4) Return to starting position.
Suggested repetitions: 3–5 with each leg.

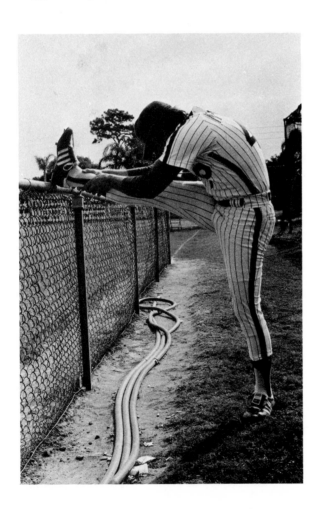

Pre-Game Warm-ups

The flexibility routines described above should be part of your daily "off-court" workout. It is designed to accomplish a specific dimension of your overall conditioning plan—the same as your endurance and strength development activities. Normally, you will not find it practical or convenient to go through this routine prior to your game of tennis, basketball or volleyball. However, some pre-game warm-ups and stretching are necessary if you're going to play your best game and avoid injury.

I'll recommend specific warm-ups and exercises for each sports category, but there is a pretty good warm-up plan that works quite well for all sports.

Begin with the warm-up activities recommended as part of your daily flexibility workout. These would include:

1. Two minutes of running in place of jogging.
2. Flexing and stretching of arms, hands, wrists and fingers.
3. Small-to-large arm circles.
4. The first 4 flexibility exercises described in this chapter.
5. Joseph Zohar recommends duplicating the various swimming strokes to get the upper body loose and warmed up. Simulate the crawl, breaststroke, backstroke and butterfly. Do each until the first suggestion of fatigue begins to be felt.
6. Spend a minute or two duplicating the various moves and strokes that you'll be using in your game—for example, forehand, backhand, volly for tennis players.

Cool-down After Workout of Game

A gradual cessation of rigorous activity is just as important as warming up before it. In order to allow your heart and lungs to recover, walk around the court, swinging the arms and rotating the shoulders and hips for 4–6 minutes. This will help your pulse rate, respiration and body temperature to gradually reduce. It is very important not to stop or sit down immediately after your game.

CHAPTER 4

Endurance

The Bottom Line

In practical terms, endurance is the "bottom line" for most sports. The weekend tennis player finds this out in very dramatic ways, especially when playing against a player with equal, or even slightly inferior, skills who is in superior physical condition. The hiker with a 35-pound pack can have his lack of conditioning brought home to him rather forcefully when his heart begins pounding, his chest starts heaving and his legs just won't carry him a step further. Even the golfer who is in poor condition is likely to notice his game coming apart on the back nine on a hot, humid day. The power drains from his legs, his grip weakens and even his coordination and confidence begin to disappear with the ebbing away of vigor.

Endurance is the ability of the body to perform rigorous physical activity for prolonged periods of time, to defer "oxygen debt," to function without fatigue. The need for optimum endurance is important to the weekend athlete for two reasons:

1. He can indulge in his sport safely without placing undue stress on his heart, if he has endurance.
2. He will play his sport better, make more shots, have more fun, win more matches; and he will be able to play more frequently and for longer periods of time, if he has endurance.

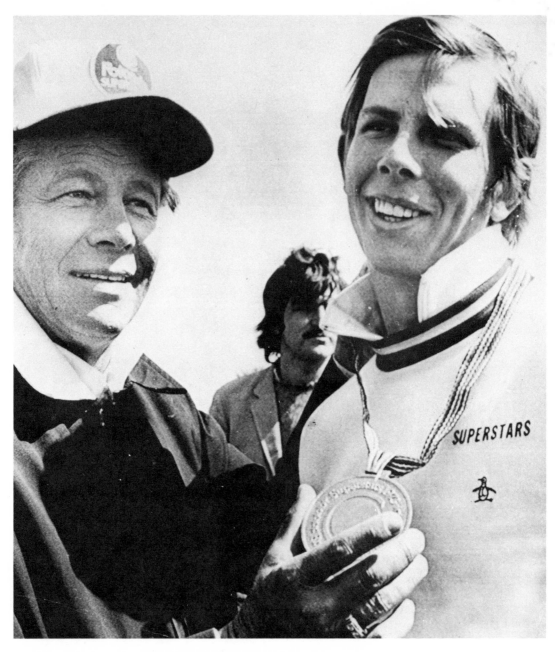

Former New York Football Gaints Star Stan Kyle Rote, Sr. congratulates "Super Star" son.
(UPI)

Professional athletes and their coaches focus on endurance as one of the major components of success on the field. Most of us have heard coaches appraise less skillful teams that are consistent winners by saying: "They're not that good, they just wear you down."

Here is what tennis star Billie Jean King says about endurance: "Fitness and conditioning become increasingly important to the tennis player as skill improves. This is because, in order to make the shot, you've got to be able to get to the ball. Two elements of conditioning come into play here: endurance and agility. Both of these elements of fitness can be improved upon. This improvement calls for a physical-training program—a program that enables a player to keep his or her game strong right up to the last point of a match, even on a hot, humid day. You've got to build endurance with a running program and regularly perform the drills that improve speed, agility and footwork."

Billie Jean's advice is certainly as meaningful to the weekend tennis player as it is to the competitive player.

Kyle Rote, Jr., by winning ABC's "Superstars Championship," demonstrated that he is as close to being the totally conditioned athlete as one can get, short of winning the Decathlon Gold Medal in the Olympics. Kyle, who plays professional soccer, has ultimate respect for endurance. He says: "My overall plan regarding conditioning is to maintain a baseline of cardio-vascular fitness [endurance] all the time, no matter what part of the season I'm in. Back in the days when I was in high school and college, we did nothing at certain times, then went overboard. We got ourselves in absolutely great shape for the football season or the basketball season, then allowed ourselves to slip into absolutely horrible shape during the summer. Luckily, we were young enough and active enough to get away with it."

"My baseline now," continued Kyle, "is running several miles a day and doing flexibility exercises every day—and that's all year long, including weekends. Some kind of routine like this is most important to the weekend athlete."

Testing—Where Am I?

Many people who decide to condition themselves for sports are already adequately motivated. Playing a respectable game of tennis is a *reason* to work out. Being able to enjoy a weekend on a mountain hiking trail with your friends or your children or your grandchildren is a *reason* to work toward cardio-respiratory fitness and strong legs.

If you accept the proposition that it is necessary to embark on a conditioning program as a pre-condition to playing active sports, the logical question for you to ask yourself is, "Where am I—in terms of my actual and potential fitness?" An important question. Consider the former athlete. He or she may still retain the self-image of ten or twenty years ago. The memories of the prime years die hard, and sometimes inactivity takes an almost unnoticed toll.

Danny Whalen, the New York Knicks trainer, made a discerning observation on this kind of situation. "One of the great hazards of rigorous sports," advises Whalen, "lies with the man or woman who may have been an outstanding high school athlete...a fine tennis player, basketball player or a track and field star. Ten or fifteen years later, this person may still regard himself or herself as a top performer—someone who has never walked away from a challenge. Suppose that challenge should come at a party, after a few too many cocktails?

"The former star athlete may readily commit to a game of tennis or handball singles or full court basketball the next day with younger or better conditioned competition. Pride may force this person to follow through and he'll probably play as though it were the NBA playoffs just to show those kids he can still do it! This person could be heading for a hospital bed—or worse." Kyle Rote, Jr., adds, "Unfortunately, people who were once athletes still have that competitive instinct. If they're playing tennis, they still want to hit that hard serve, they still want to chase down every ball and they still want to run around in the sun like everyone else. This can be a very dangerous situation."

On the other hand, there are many people for whom sports activity is a brand new idea. They will find out very quickly that sports such as volleyball, skiing or any of the racquet sports are very taxing and will leave them stiff, sore and exhausted. The right fitness program can make these, and all sports, more fun and a lot safer.

Fitness Tests

How does one find out what his state of fitness is? The first step is a visit to your physician. Tell him that you are planning to undertake a conditioning program and ask him to help you determine your present state of fitness. This is especially important if you are over thirty-five years old, are more than fifteen percent overweight, are a heavy smoker or have any history of serious illness or injury. Part of your physical examination will be an electrocardiogram, usually referred to as an EKG. It is highly advisable to have your physician arrange that you be given a "stress" EKG, which describes the efficiency of the heart under conditions of physical exertion. You can show him the walk-jog test described in this chapter and, with his permission, use that method to determine your fitness level.

You may wish to have a professional evaluation made of your state of fitness. You will be surprised at how easy it is to have a complete test done by a fitness expert. Practically every YMCA and YWCA has the necessary equipment and personnel with the expertise to provide you with a total fitness profile including body composition (body fat vs. muscle tissue), circulatory-respiratory fitness, strength and flexibility. The Y's also can include you in a supervised, customized fitness program which will help you overcome your fitness shortcomings.

Circulatory-respiratory fitness is the component usually associated with the quality we call *endurance*. It is a function of how well the body can process oxygen and transport it to the tissues. At the same time—as a reciprocal action—carbon monoxide and other by-products of muscular activity must be carried from the tissues through the circulatory-respiratory system and exhaled. The efficiency of the circulatory-respiratory system can be measured quite accurately and is expressed in terms of milliliters of oxygen processed per kilogram of body weight per minute. For short, we call this "aerobic" capacity, using the term invented and popularized by Kenneth H. Cooper, M.D., who pioneered in the development of circulatory-respiratory fitness for the layman.

I have provided a test which can be self-administered, a test geared to comfortable performance and perfect for the non-conditioned or moderately conditioned person.

A Fitness Test You Can Do Yourself

The President's Council on Physical Fitness and Sports has devised a simple test which measures cardio-vascular fitness. If you are a newcomer to physical fitness, this self-test will indicate a starter program just right for your capacity. If your physician has given you the green light, you're ready to begin.

The tests described here will measure your present exercise tolerance, which determines where you start in the walking-jogging part of your endurance program. Exercise capacity varies widely among individuals, even when they are similar in age and physical build. That's why your program should be based on your personal test results rather than on what someone else is doing or on what you think you should be able to do.

WALK TEST

The object of this test is to determine how many minutes (up to 10) you can walk at a brisk pace, without undue difficulty or discomfort, on a level surface.

—If you cannot walk for 5 minutes, you should begin with the Red walking program in this chapter.

—If you can walk more than 5 minutes, but less than 10, you should begin with the third week of the Red walking program.

—If you can walk for the full 10 minutes, but are somewhat tired and sore as a result, you should start with the White walking-jogging program.

—If you can breeze through the full 10 minutes, you are ready for bigger things. Wait until the next day and take the Walk-Jog Test.

WALK-JOG TEST

In this test, you alternately walk 50 steps (left foot strikes the ground 25 times) and jog 50 steps for a total of 10 minutes. Read the jogging guidelines later in this chapter before taking the test.

Walk at the rate of 120 steps per minute (left foot strikes the ground at 1-second intervals). Jog at the rate of 144 steps per minute (left foot strikes ground 18 times every 15 seconds).

—If you cannot complete the 10-minute test, begin at the third week of the White Program.

—If you can complete the 10-minute test, but are tired and winded as a result, start with the last week of the White Program before moving on to the Blue Program.

—If you perform the 10-minute test without difficulty, start with the Blue Program.

A word of caution: If, during these tests, you experience nausea, trembling, extreme breathlessness, pounding in the head or pain in the chest, stop immediately. If the symptoms persist beyond the point of temporary discomfort, check with your physician.

The symptoms described are signs that you have reached the limits of your present exercise tolerance. The point at which they begin to occur indicates where you should start in the exercise program.

Other Indicators

LISTEN TO YOUR BODY

Many readers will accept the need for fitness rather more easily than they will accommodate to the regimented fitness formulas. Dr. George Sheehan not only understands such people, he identifies with them. "It's a matter of listening to your body," says Dr. Sheehan. "If you put someone on a stress machine and tell him to go at mild exertion, he will. He'll go at just about fifty percent of his VO max (maximum oxygen utilization). Look," he points out, "you've never heard of a horse running himself to death without a jockey on his back." Dr. Sheehan makes a very strong point of something that is easy to overlook: *If your body tells you you're straining, don't challenge it!*

THE TALK TEST

Sometimes books like this tend to make simple things complicated. In a moment of welcome clarity, I came upon some advice by one of the country's foremost authorities on fitness and conditioning, William J. Bowerman. A professor of physical education, a track coach and author of *Jogging,* one of the most influential publications on conditioning for the layman, Bowerman has pin-pointed the basic test for anyone engaged in a conditioning program. He calls it the "talk test." It simply means that anyone in a conditioning program—no matter what their level—should be able to converse with a companion. If you're too winded to be able to speak, you've exceeded your aerobic capacity. It's that simple.

Increase Your Oxygen Uptake

The best way to understand an individual's circulatory-respiratory endurance or aerobic capacity is to measure his ability to process oxygen (milliliters of oxygen, per kilogram per minute), or his ml./kg./min. Most people who deal with fitness on a professional level call this "oxygen uptake." The higher the maximum oxygen uptake is for an individual, the better the shape of his oxygen processing machinery. You may be able to process oxygen at a rate of 35–40 ml./kg./min. if you are in average shape or perhaps up to 45–55 ml./kg./min. if you are in reasonably good condition. Some of the great milers, such as Marty Liquori and Jim Ryun—athletes whose oxygen demands are enormous—have measured in the area of 80 to 85 milliliters of oxygen per kilogram per minute. In other words, these athletes possess circulatory-respiratory systems roughly two hundred percent more efficient than the average weekend athlete's.

The way in which we increase our cardio-respiratory endurance is by means of a carefully planned, carefully followed conditioning program. Such a program has far-reaching effects on the body—transcending the obvious benefits to the heart and lungs. In *The Physical Fitness Research Digest,* published and distributed by the President's Council on Physical Fitness and Sports, cardio-respiratory endurance is described as "contractions of large muscle groups for relatively long periods of time, during which maximal adjustments of the circulatory-respiratory system to the activity are necessary, such as in distance running and swimming." This publication goes on to say that the elements involved are "the heart, the vessels supplying blood to all parts of the body, the oxygen-carrying capacity of that blood, and the capillary system receiving that blood."

What all this means is that once you get a physical-fitness program in gear that can provide positive improvement and a training effect to the cardio-respiratory system, a lot of other good things are happening to you. You'll probably sleep better, be less frequently troubled by minor health problems such as headaches, heartburn, indigestion and nervous disorders. In other words, it's difficult to be "shaped up for sports" and still be unhealthy in any other dimension—aside from disease or other outside influences—since your conditioning activities are feeding oxygen-rich blood regularly to all the organs of the body.

Some Basic Endurance Programs

"Running is the most important part of my conditioning program," says Major League pitcher Tug McGraw. "I run," says NFL great Paul Warfield, "to maintain overall fitness. It is the best conditioner and body builder I have tried." "During the off season, I run," confides LPGA golfer, Laura Baugh. With very few exceptions, most of the world's best professional athletes and top amateurs have made running the keystone of their conditioning programs. One reason that running apparently is the universal prescription is that, by making the appropriate adjustments in intensity, duration and frequency, it can be made to suit just about anyone's fitness requirements.

There are some other very effective endurance activities, such as rope skipping and cycling, which we will cover later in this chapter. Running, however, is a convenient method for most people to train, so let's see how best to approach it.

RUNNING AND JOGGING GUIDELINES

Paul Warfield has been chasing and catching passes in the National Football League for several years. He's a runner and he advises: "Avoid common bad habits in running form. Don't run 'tight'—that is, don't tense the muscles in your arms, shoulders and upper body. Concentrate on swinging your arms easily and running with curled, but not clenched hands. This will help you develop a fluid style and a more efficient stride." In order to develop a permanent conditioning program based on running, it has to become pleasurable for you. And it can, if you follow Paul's advice and run *loose*. Running is one of mankind's primal activities; we were meant to run. You would never know it to observe some of the weekend joggers chugging along the nation's highways and footpaths, arms pumping, fists clenched, faces contorted and puffing and wheezing like steam engines. This is not training—it is straining. Learn to run loose . . . relax . . . glide . . . stride. Do this for a short distance, if that's all you are capable of. Then, gradually increase distance.

Here are some jogging tips developed by the President's Council on Physical Fitness and Sports:

- Run in an upright position, avoiding the tendency to lean. Keep your back as straight as you can and still remain comfortable. Keep your head up; don't watch your feet.
- Hold arms slightly away from body, with elbows bent so that the forearms are approximately parallel to the ground. Occasionally, shaking and relaxing the arms and shoulders will help reduce the tightness that sometimes develops while

jogging. Periodically taking several deep breaths and blowing them out completely also will help you to relax.

- It is best to land on the heel of the foot and rock forward, so that you drive off the ball of the foot for your next step. If this proves difficult, try a more flat-footed style. Jogging on the balls of the feet only, as in sprinting, will produce severe soreness in the legs.

- Keep steps short, letting the foot strike the ground beneath the knee instead of reaching out to the front. Length of stride should vary with your rate of speed.

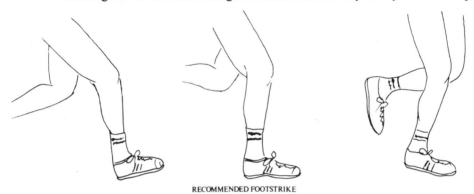

RECOMMENDED FOOTSTRIKE

WHAT TO WEAR

Select loose, comfortable clothes. Dress for warmth in the winter, coolness in the summer. "Jogging suits" or "warm-ups" are not necesssary, but they are extremely practical and comfortable, and they can help to create a commitment to jogging.

Do not wear rubberized or plastic clothing. Increased sweating will not produce permanent weight loss, and such clothing can cause body temperatures to rise to dangerous levels. They interfere with evaporation of perspiration, which is the body's chief temperature-control mechanism during exercise. If perspiration cannot evaporate, heat stroke or heat exhaustion may result.

Properly fitting shoes with firm soles, good arch supports and pliable tops are essential. Shoes made especially for distance running or walking are recommended. Ripple or crepe soles are excellent for running on hard surfaces. Beginners should avoid inexpensive, thin-soled sneakers. Wear clean, soft, heavy, well-fitting socks. You may want to wear thin socks under the heavier pair. Additional information on footwear will be found in the chapter dealing with "Sports Injuries."

WHERE TO JOG

If possible, avoid hard surfaces such as asphalt and concrete. Running tracks (located at most high schools), grass playing fields, parks and golf courses are recommended. In inclement weather, jog in church, school or YMCA gymnasiums; in protected areas around shopping centers; or in your garage or basement. Varying locations and routes will add interest to your program.

WHEN TO JOG

The time of day is not important, although it is best not to jog during the first hour after eating, or during the middle of a hot, humid day. The important thing is to commit yourself to a regular schedule. Some believe that people who jog in the morning tend to be more faithful than those who run in the evenings. Persons who jog with family members or friends also tend to adhere to their schedules better. However, companionship—not competition—should be your motive when jogging with someone else.

Endurance—Starter Program

If you've taken the walk test or the walk-jog test described in chapter 1, you'll know exactly where to begin your endurance-starter program. This program or a similar one is a *must* for the inactive person contemplating any fast-moving sports activity such as tennis, squash, racquet ball, handball, volleyball or any of the endurance activities such as hiking or backpacking. I can't stress this too strongly. You'll get much more pleasure from your tennis game if you get your flexibility and endurance programs well underway before you begin to play. Try to achieve at least the fourth week of the Blue Program before beginning your sport. It is truly a worthwhile investment.

WARM-UP FIRST

Before this endurance program or any conditioning activities are attempted, the body should be warmed up to increase respiration and body temperature, to stretch ligaments and connective tissue. Refer to the "Warm-up" chapter of this book.

RED—WALKING PROGRAM

Daily Activity

Week 1: Walk at a brisk pace for 5 minutes, or for a shorter period if you become uncomfortably tired. Walk slowly or rest for three minutes. Again walk briskly for 5 minutes or until you become uncomfortably tired.

Week 2: Same as Week 1, but increase pace as soon as you can walk 5 minutes without soreness or fatigue.

Week 3: Walk at a brisk pace for 8 minutes, or for a shorter time if you become uncomfortably tired. Walk slowly or rest for 3 minutes. Again walk briskly for 8 minutes, or until you become uncomfortably tired.

Week 4: Same as Week 3, but increase pace as soon as you can walk 8 minutes without soreness or fatigue.

When you have completed Week 4 of the Red Program, begin at Week 1 of the White Program.

WHITE—WALKING-JOGGING PROGRAM

Daily Activity

Week 1: Walk at a brisk pace for 10 minutes, or for a shorter period of time if you become uncomfortably tired. Walk slowly or rest for 3 minutes. Again walk briskly for 10 minutes, or until you become uncomfortably tired.

Week 2: Walk at a brisk pace for 15 minutes, or for a shorter time if you become uncomfortably tired. Walk slowly for 3 minutes.

Week 3: Jog 10 seconds (25 yards). Walk 1 minute (100 yards). Repeat 12 times.

Week 4: Jog 20 seconds (50 yards). Walk 1 minute (100 yards). Repeat 12 times.

When you have completed Week 4 of the White Program, begin at Week 1 of the Blue Program.

BLUE—JOGGING PROGRAM

Daily Activity

Week 1: Jog 40 seconds (100 yards). Walk 1 minute (100 yards). Repeat 9 times.

Week 2: Jog 1 minute (150 yards). Walk 1 minute (100 yards). Repeat 8 times.

Week 3: Jog 2 minutes (300 yards). Walk 1 minute (100 yards). Repeat 6 times.

Week 4: Jog 4 minutes (600 yards). Walk 1 minute (100 yards). Repeat 4 times.

Week 5: Jog 6 minutes (900 yards). Walk 1 minute (100 yards). Repeat 3 times.

Week 6: Jog 8 minutes (1,200 yards). Walk 2 minutes (200 yards). Repeat 2 times.

Week 7: Jog 10 minutes (1,500 yards). Walk 2 minutes (200 yards). Repeat 2 times.

Week 8: Jog 12 minutes (1,700 yards). Walk 2 minutes (200 yards). Repeat 2 times.

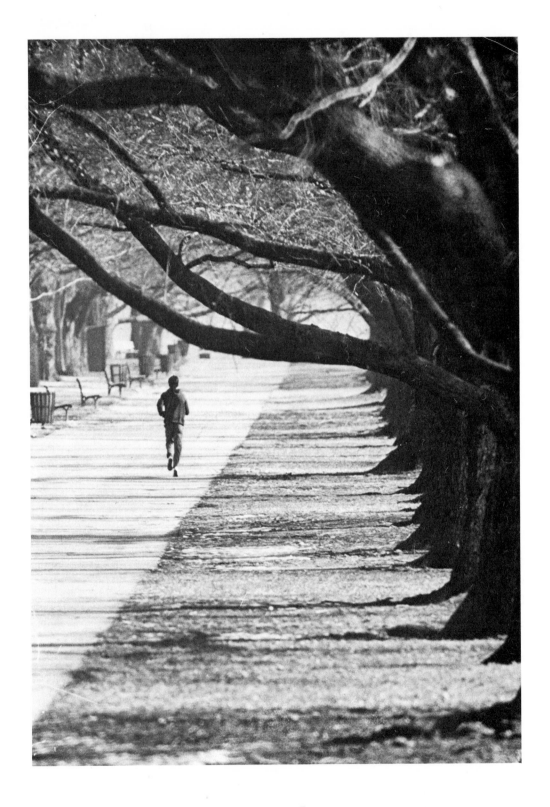

Intermediate Program (Jog-Run)

Now that you've progressed through the Blue jogging program, you're beginning to have an appreciation of what fitness and conditioning are all about. You're feeling better than you've felt in a long time—maybe better than you've ever felt. Now you're ready for a brisk round of tennis on the weekend; you can handle it, at least in terms of endurance. But don't stop now. You're in better shape than you were, but you're not in great shape. That elusive goal is really not that far away, though. Just twelve weeks, if you follow this intermediate jogging-running program. Is it worth it? Think back to how you used to feel. Once again Paul Warfield has something relevant to say about the subject: "Most people, and even athletes in less physically demanding sports, go through life without even knowing what it's like to be physically fit. It is a joy, indeed, to experience a true feeling of fitness, and to find self-expression through it. Most people indulge in a moderate amount of exercise, but very few get even a glimpse of true fitness or find out what it feels like to be a complete person."

That's an exciting picture that Paul Warfield paints and you can make it a self-portrait, if you pursue it. The next step—and the biggest—is this intermediate program.*

You're Ready

If you've followed the starter program or if you are already reasonably active, you're ready for the Intermediate Program. You're able to jog 1 mile slowly without undue fatigue, rest 2 minutes, and do it again. Your sessions consume about 250 calories.

You're ready to increase both the intensity and the duration of your runs. You'll be using the heart-rate training zone for those of medium fitness (35–45 ml./kg./min.). You'll begin jogging 1 mile in 12 minutes, and when you finish this program, you may be able to complete 3 or more miles at a pace approaching 8 minutes a mile. Each week's program includes three phases: (1) the basic workout, (2) longer runs (overdistance) and (3) shorter runs (underdistance). If a week's program seems too easy, move ahead; if it seems too hard, move back a week or two. Remember—a warm-up and a cool-down must be part of each exercise session.

---

* This program was developed by Brian J. Sharkey, director of Human Performance Laboratory, University of Montana. It originally appeared in *Fitness and Work Capacity* U.S. Dept. of Agriculture Publication No. 7661 2811.

PACE GUIDE FOR GAUGING SPEED OVER VARIOUS DISTANCES

	Pace	1 Mile	½ Mile	¼ Mile	220 Yards	100 Yards	50 Yards
				(in minutes and seconds)			
Slow jog	10 cal./min. (120 cal./mile)*	12:00	6:00	3:00	1:30	0:40	0:20
Jog	12 cal./min. (120 cal./mile)*	10:00	5:00	2:30	1:15	0:34	0:17
Run	15 cal./min. (120 cal./mile)*	8:00	4:00	2:00	1:00	0:27	0:13
Fast run	20 cal./min. (120 cal./mile)*	6:00	3:00	1:30	0:45	0:20	0:10

*Depends on efficiency and body size; add 10 percent for each 15 pounds over 150; subtract 10 percent for each 15 pounds under 150.

Week 1

Basic Workout (Monday, Thursday):
 1 mile in 11 minutes; active recovery (walk). Run twice.

Underdistance (Tuesday, Friday):
 ¼ mile to ½ mile slowly.
 ½ mile in 5 minutes 30 seconds. Run twice (recover between repeats).
 ¼ mile in 2 minutes 45 seconds. Run 4 times (recover between repeats).
 Jog ¼ to ½ mile slowly.

Overdistance (Wednesday, Saturday or Sunday):
 2 miles slowly. (Use the talk test: Jog at a pace that allows you to converse.)

Week 2

Basic Workout (Monday, Thursday):
 1 mile in 10 minutes 30 seconds; active recovery. Run twice.

Underdistance (Tuesday, Friday):
 ¼ to ½ mile slowly.
 ½ mile in 5 minutes.
 ¼ mile in 2 minutes 30 seconds. Run 2 times (recover between repeats).
 ¼ mile in 2 minutes 45 seconds. Run 2 times (recover between repeats).
 220 yards in 1 minute 20 seconds. Run 4 times (recover between repeats).
 ¼ to ½ mile slowly.

Overdistance (Wednesday, Saturday or Sunday):
   2¼ miles slowly.

WEEK 3

Basic Workout (Monday, Thursday):
   1 mile in 10 minutes, active recovery. Run twice.

Underdistance (Tuesday, Friday):
   ¼ to ½ mile slowly.
   ½ mile in 4 minutes 45 seconds.
   ¼ mile in 2 minutes 30 seconds. Run 4 times (recover between repeats).
   220 yards in 30 seconds. Run 4 times (recover between repeats).
   100 yards in 30 seconds. Run 4 times (recover between repeats).
   ¼ to ½ mile slowly.

Overdistance:
   2½ miles slowly.

WEEK 4

Basic Workout (Monday, Thursday):
   1 mile in 9 minutes 30 seconds; active recovery. Run twice.

Underdistance (Tuesday, Friday):
   ¼ to ½ mile slowly.
   ½ mile in 4 minutes 45 seconds.
   ¼ mile in 2 minutes 20 seconds. Run 4 times (recover between repeats).
   220 yards in 1 minute. Run 4 times (recover between repeats).
   ¼ to ½ mile slowly.

Overdistance (Wednesday, Saturday or Sunday):
   2¾ miles slowly.

WEEK 5

Basic Workout (Monday, Thursday):
   1 mile in 9 minutes; active recovery. Run twice.

Underdistance (Tuesday, Friday):
   ¼ to ½ mile slowly.
   ½ mile in 4 minutes 30 seconds.
   ¼ mile in 2 minutes 20 seconds. Run 4 times (recover between repeats).

220 yards in 60 seconds. Run 4 times (recover between repeats).
100 yards in 27 seconds. Run 4 times (Recover between repeats).
¼ to ½ mile slowly.

Overdistance (Wednesday, Saturday or Sunday):
3 miles slowly.

WEEK 6

Basic Workout (Monday, Thursday):
1½ miles in 13 minutes 30 seconds; active recovery. Run twice.

Underdistance (Tuesday, Friday):
¼ to ½ mile slowly.
½ mile in 4 minutes 30 seconds. Run twice (recover between repeats).
¼ mile in 2 minutes 10 seconds. Run 4 times (recover between repeats).
220 yards in 60 seconds. Run 4 times (recover between repeats).
100 yards in 25 seconds. Run twice (recover between repeats).
¼ to ½ mile slowly.

Overdistance (Wednesday, Saturday or Sunday):
3 miles slowly; INCREASE PACE last ½ mile.

WEEK 7

Basic Workout (Monday, Thursday):
1½ miles in 13 minutes; active recovery. Run twice.

Underdistance (Tuesday, Friday):
¼ to ½ mile slowly.
½ mile in 4 minutes 15 seconds. Run twice (recover between repeats).
¼ mile in 2 minutes. Run 4 times (recover between repeats).
220 yards in 55 seconds. Run 4 times (recover between repeats).
¼ to ½ mile slowly.

Overdistance (Wednesday, Saturday or Sunday):
3½ miles slowly; always increase pace near finish.

WEEK 8

Basic Workout (Monday, Thursday):
1 mile in 8 minutes; active recovery; run 1 mile in 8 minutes 30 seconds; active recovery; repeat (total of 3 miles).

Underdistance (Tuesday, Friday):
  ¼ to ½ mile slowly.
  ½ mile in 4 minutes. Run twice (recover between repeats).
  ¼ mile in 1 minute 50 seconds. Run 4 times (recover between repeats).
  220 yards in 55 seconds. Run 4 times (recover between repeats).
  100 yards in 23 seconds. Run 4 times (recover between repeats).
  ¼ to ½ mile slowly.

Overdistance (Wednesday, Saturday or Sunday):
  3¾ miles slowly.

WEEK 9

Basic Workout (Monday, Thursday):
  1 mile in 8 minutes. Run 3 times (recover between repeats).

Underdistance (Tuesday, Friday):
  ¼ to ½ mile slowly.
  ½ mile in 3 minutes 30 seconds.
  ¼ mile in 1 minute 45 seconds. Run 4 times (recover between repeats).
  220 yards in 50 seconds. Run 4 times (recover between repeats).
  100 yards in 20 seconds. Run 4 times (recover between repeats).
  50 yards in 10 seconds. Run 4 times (recover between repeats).
  ¼ to ½ mile slowly.

Overdistance (Wednesday, Saturday or Sunday):
  4 miles slowly.

WEEK 10

Basic Workout (Monday, Thursday):
  1½ miles in 12 minutes. Run twice (recover between repeats).

Underdistance (Tuesday, Friday):
  ¼ to ½ mile slowly.
  ½ mile in 3 minutes 45 seconds. Run 3 times (recover between repeats).
  ¼ mile in 1 minute 50 seconds. Run 6 times (recover between repeats).
  220 yards in 45 seconds. Run twice (recover between repeats).
  ¼ to ½ mile slowly.

Overdistance (Wednesday, Saturday or Sunday):
  4 miles; increase pace last ½ mile.

Week 11

Basic Workout (Monday, Thursday):
  1 mile in 7 minutes 30 seconds. Run 3 times (recover between repeats).

Underdistance (Tuesday, Friday):
  ¼ to ½ mile slowly.
  ½ mile in 3 minutes 50 seconds. Run 4 times (recover between repeats).
  ¼ mile in 1 minute 45 seconds. Run 4 times (recover between repeats).
  220 yards in 45 seconds. Run 2 times (recover between repeats).
  ¼ to ½ mile slowly.

Overdistance (Wednesday, Saturday or Sunday):
  Over 4 miles slowly (more than 400 calories per workout).

Week 12

Basic Workout:
  1½ miles in 11 minutes 40 seconds.

You've achieved the fitness standard of 45 ml./kg./min. Proceed to the advanced aerobic fitness program.

Advanced Aerobic Training

This section is for the well-trained runner. I'll provide some suggestions for advanced training, but keep in mind there is no single way to train. If you enjoy underdistance training, by all means use it. If you find that you prefer overdistance, you'll like the suggestions offered here.

Long, slow distance running seems to be the ideal way to train. It combines the features of over- and underdistance with a minimum of discomfort. Simply pick up the pace as you approach the end of a long run, and you'll receive an optimal training stimulus. Moreover, since the speed work is limited to a short span near the end of the run, discomfort is brief.

Consider the following suggestions:

- Always warm-up before your run.
- Use the high fitness heart-rate training zone.
- Vary the location and distance of the run (long-short; fast-slow; hilly-flat).

- Set distance goals:

  Phase 1:   20 miles a week.

  Phase 2:   25 miles a week (ready for 3–5-mile road races).

  Phase 3:   30 miles a week.

  Phase 4:   35 miles a week (ready for 5–7-mile road races).

  Phase 5:   40 miles a week.

  Phase 6:   45 miles a week (ready for 7–10-mile road races).

  Phase 7:   More than 50 miles a week (consider longer races, such as the Marathon—26.2 miles).

- Don't be a slave to your goals, and don't increase weekly mileage unless you enjoy it.
- Run 6 days a week, if you enjoy it; otherwise try an alternate-day schedule with longer runs.
- Try one long run (not over one-third of weekly distance) on Saturday or Sunday.
- Try two shorter runs, if the long ones seem difficult: 5 + 5 instead of 10.
- Keep records, if you like—you'll be surprised! Record date, distance, comments. Note resting and work pulse, body weight. Every six weeks check your performance over a measured distance to observe progress (use a local road race or the 1½-mile-run test). Check your fitness score on the step test several times a year.
- Don't train with a stopwatch. Wear a wristwatch, so you'll know how long you've run.
- Increase speed as you approach the finish of a run.
- Always cool down after a run.

Alternative Endurance Activities

Rope Skipping

Many athletes have told me that they use rope skipping as a conditioner as an alternative to running, especially when they are traveling. Professional golfers, particularly, are becoming boosters of the skipping rope as a training device. It is truly a portable gym. It can be carried anywhere and used anywhere. Golfers on the Pro Tour often skip rope in their hotel rooms during the golf season, since their travel schedules do not readily accommodate the usual training procedures. Laura Baugh, who plays the Women's Tour said: "Running is my basic conditioner. It's important that a golfer keep the leg muscles toned and keep his or her endurance up. I skip rope each evening in the hotel when I'm on the tour. Several hundred repetitions daily replaces my running program when I'm traveling."

Rope skipping is becoming almost a standard conditioning activity for tennis players. Billie Jean King and Stan Smith have encouraged rope skipping as a training technique for young tennis players. Skipping rope not only builds cardio-vascular endurance but it develops "fast feet" or agility. Additionally, this exercise sharpens coordination—the interaction between the eyes, hands and arms, feet and legs.

When you begin skipping rope, you may find it to be a difficult activity. It will probably take you a few days to get into the swing of it.

It is important that your rope be long enough. If the rope is too short, you're going to be continually tripping over it. You can tell if it is long enough by standing on it with both feet. The ends should be able to reach your armpits. Commercial ropes are available with swivels or ball bearings in the handles. These ropes are easier to use and are less likely to kink.

ROPE SKIPPING AS INTERVAL CONDITIONER

Rope skipping is an effective form of conditioning, although for most weekend athletes it is not a recommended form of regular exercise. The demands made on the cardio-respiratory system are severe and can be accelerated very quickly. Ten minutes of rope skipping can be equivalent to 20–30 minutes of jogging. The danger lies in the possibility of the heart rate climbing rapidly into dangerous areas. You may find that rope skipping is a good "rainy-day" conditioner if you use it as an interval-training technique. Here's how. Skip rope until you feel the onset of fatigue or breathlessness (this may be only 30 seconds or so), then stop. Rest until you recover (about 1 minute), then skip again. Do *not* allow yourself to skip until extremely winded. Be moderate!

If you are in fairly good shape now, perhaps well into the Intermediate Jog-Run Program, you may want to use this twelve-week rope-skipping program as an alternative. If it makes too much of a demand on you, decrease the jumping time slightly and increase the rest interval, until you can handle the first level of the program as outlined. You will probably be able to progress from there, using the program guidelines.

12-Week Rope-Skipping Program

Jump, rest 60 seconds and jump again; 3 times during each workout using the following schedule:

Week	Skip	Week	Skip
1	30 Seconds	7	2 minutes
2	45 seconds	8	2 minutes, 15 seconds
3	1 minute	9	2 minutes, 30 seconds
4	1 minute, 15 seconds	10	2 minutes, 45 seconds
5	1 minute, 30 seconds	11	3 minutes
6	1 minute, 45 seconds	12	3 minutes, 25 seconds

After three months of rope skipping, your cardio-vascular fitness will be greatly improved, your leg strength and muscular endurance will be dramatically improved and you will be surprised at your increased agility and coordination. You can now proceed to up to 8–10 minutes of skipping maintaining the 60-second rest intervals. To make your skipping sessions more fun, you can experiment with a variety of steps and rhythms.

Rope Skipping Not for Everyone

It should be stressed that rope skipping is not recommended for everyone. Some people—especially those who carry a large amount of weight or who have structural defects of the feet—may experience a great deal of discomfort, not to mention outright injury of the feet. Rope skipping requires the jumper to land on the balls of the feet, putting considerable stress on the metatarsal area. The rolling heel-to-toe footstrike that absorbs the pounding of foot against ground for the jogger is not possible when skipping rope. If you experience pain while skipping rope, stop! Find another conditioning method before you inflict severe injury to your feet.

Some sports physicians are recommending that rope skipping be reserved for periods of bad weather or during travel, when outside jogging is not possible or convenient, rather than as a regular conditioning activity.

STATIONARY CYCLING

Many gyms are equipped with stationary cycles. You can obtain one for your home at a reasonable cost (around $100). Training with a cycle can even be fun if you set it up in front of your television set or hi-fi. It is absolutely mandatory that your cycle have a device to control the resistance to your cycling effort.

Begin pedaling at an even pace with moderate resistance for 5 minutes, get off your cycle and walk easily for 1 minute, pedal again for 5 minutes. That's your sequence: pedal, rest 1 minute, pedal. Build up your endurance, as follows:

Week 1: pedal 5 minutes.
Week 2: pedal 6 minutes.
Week 3: pedal 7 minutes.
Week 4: pedal 8 minutes.
Week 5: pedal 9 minutes.

Begin the sixth week of cycling by pedaling at a brisk pace with moderate resistance for 10 minutes. Get off your cycle and walk easily for 1 minute, pedal again for 10 minutes. Build up to a single 30-minute session as follows:

Week 7: pedal 12 minutes.
Week 8: pedal 15 minutes.
Week 9: pedal 18 minutes.
Week 10: pedal 20 minutes.
Week 11: pedal 25 minutes.
Week 12: pedal 30 minutes.

After three months of endurance cycling, increase the duration of pedaling as time and your physical progress allow; or better yet, get yourself a bicycle and get into an outdoor endurance cycling program.

RUNNING THE TREADMILL

For some of us, this exercise may have philosophical and psychological overtones that cause us either to smile and get on with it or perhaps look around for another fitness method. Assuming that one is not already on a perpetual treadmill, this is a pretty effective indoor conditioning activity. A treadmill is not normally considered an at-home type of conditioning apparatus. A good one is fairly expensive, but most Y's, health clubs and fitness centers have them, since they are often part of the standard aerobic testing equipment. If you have access to a treadmill and would like to use it as an aerobic conditioning device or when running outdoors is not feasible, here is a program that progresses at about the same rate as the jogging and rope-skipping programs already described.

Begin the first week by walking on the treadmill at a brisk pace for 5 minutes. Rest for 3 minutes. Walk for 5 minutes. Gradually lengthen walking period, maintaining the 3-minute resting period between walks (walk, rest 3 minutes, walk) as follows:

Week 2: walk 5 minutes 30 seconds.
Week 3: walk 6 minutes.
Week 4: walk 7 minutes.
Week 5: walk 8 minutes.

Begin the sixth week by walking at a brisk pace for 10 minutes, rest 3 minutes, then walk 10 minutes. Gradually build up to 15 minutes walking without fatigue. Then begin a slow, easy jog for 5 minutes, walk 3 minutes, and jog again for 6 minutes. Repeat daily (jog, rest 3 minutes, jog) until you are able to jog for two 8-minute periods.

After three months of running the treadmill, you should be able to handle continuous 30-minute running sessions. If you can, it's about time you left the confines of the gym or your basement and launched your outdoors running program. You'll have a lot more fun, you'll have access to a better supply of oxygen-rich air and you may become a serious runner.

SWEDISH WALKING PROGRAM

It is quite possible that many readers will want to try a slower, more relaxed approach to cardio-respiratory fitness. For many senior golfers, for example, a program geared to walking rather than running or jogging might be appropriate.

Recently the President's Council on Physical Fitness and Sports has endorsed the Swedish Walking Program, developed by Maryland attorney and physical-fitness enthusiast

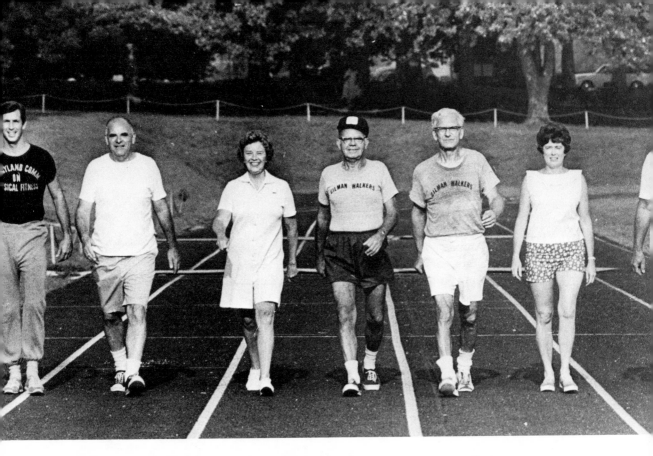

Harry D. Kaufman. As Dr. George Sheehan says, "Find your sport...find your way to physical fitness." And for a growing number of people all over America, Swedish walking is an acceptable and an appealing way to improve circulatory-respiratory fitness.

This program usually takes the form of a twelve-week supervised clinic. Such clinics, or classes, are springing up in many communities and cities throughout the country. Anyone interested in joining or starting such a class can get the relevant details from the Maryland Commission on Physical Fitness in Baltimore, Maryland.

Swedish Walking Method

The Swedish walking method is composed of five elements that make it somewhat different from just walking:

1. First of all, a heel-to-toe footstrike is recommended, just the same as the one described in the jogging section. This provides for a smooth, "rolling" action, rather than a pounding one.
2. The second area of concentration is on proper breathing. Essentially, this means deep, rhythmic breathing. Mr. Kaufman suggests that, every 100 yards or so, the walker take especially deep breaths and let them all the way out. This assures that plenty of fresh oxygen is made available to the circulatory-respiratory system.
3. Posture is important. The back should be kept reasonably straight and the head held

with the chin up, rather than pressing down toward the chest. Erect posture and high chin facilitate easy breathing.

4. Gradually, the walker is able to lengthen his stride so that, before long, he is walking briskly.
5. Finally, the one other ingredient that makes Swedish walking a conditioning method is the employment of mild stretching exercises while walking.

Some of the exercises Harry Kaufman recommends for building upper torso strength while walking are the following:

1. Extend arms in front of the body, squeeze hands into a fist, then shake fingers. Do this about 5 times.
2. Extend arms out from sides and rotate arms and shoulders through complete 360-degree circles, in both directions, 4 or 5 times.
3. Shrug shoulders up and down, forward and backward several times.
4. Thrust arms straight forward and retract them several times.
5. Thrust arms out from sides and retract them several times.

These exercises are only a sampling of the kinds of stretching activities that can be done while walking. Use your imagination and do whatever your body tells you is a worthwhile exercise. The exercises are not done constantly, but are introduced at intervals during the walking period. Here's a twelve-week program that should have anyone on the road to fitness.

12-Week Swedish Walking Program

WEEK 1

Session 1: ¾-mile slow walk.
  Concentrate on how to walk (heel to toe). Learn how to deep breathe. Learn correct body posture, including movement of arms. Give deep breathing exercises every 220 yards.
Session 2: ¾-mile slow walk.
  Same instructions as in Session 1.
Session 3: ¾-mile slow walk.
  Same instructions as in Session 1.

WEEK 2

Session 1: ⅞-mile walk.
  Start to gradually lengthen stride, varying pace, alternating slow to a medium stride. Continue deep breathing exercises and emphasize correct body posture.

Session 2: ⅞-mile walk.

Same instructions as in Session 1, week 2.

Session 3: ⅞-mile walk.

Same instructions as in Session 1, week 2.

WEEK 3

Session 1: 1-mile walk.

Again, lengthen stride. Add the additional breathing exercise, while walking, of holding in the stomach and extending the chest for short intervals. It is necessary to hold the body erect and use a step almost similar to the goose step. Continue for only 55 yards, then alternate the pace, at times slow, at times a little faster, and then yet a little faster. At this time, emphasize heel-to-toe walking, so that everybody will be walking normally with a heel-to-toe stride.

Session 2: 1-mile walk.

Same instructions as in Session 1, week 3.

Session 3: 1-mile walk.

Same instructions as in Session 1, week 3.

WEEK 4

Session 1: Distance 1⅛ miles.

Continue everything stressed in weeks 1, 2 and 3, and add for the first time exercises while walking, including shoulder and arm exercises. Gradually lengthen the stride again.

Session 2: Distance 1⅛ miles.

Same instructions as in Session 1, week 4.

Session 3: Distance 1⅛ miles.

Same instructions as in Session 1, week 4.

WEEK 5

Session 1: Walk 1¼ miles.

Continue as in week 4, but add for the first time isometric exercises while walking. Again, lengthen the stride.

Session 2: Walk 1¼ miles.

Same instructions as in Session 1, week 5.

Session 3: Walk 1¼ miles.

Same instructions as in Session 1, week 5.

Week 6

Session 1: Walk 1½ miles.
> Lengthen stride that will be the fastest pace for the course. Alternate between slow, moderate and fast, which is known as the Swedish Fartlek. Include arm and shoulder exercises.

Session 2: Walk 1½ miles.
> Add a slow trot to alternating fast and slow walking and the various-type calisthenics.

Session 3: Walk 1½ miles.
> Same instructions as in Session 2, week 6.

Week 7

Session 1: Distance 1⅝ miles.
> Walk briskly for ½ mile, then walk moderately for 220 yards; walk briskly again for ½ mile, then walk at a moderate pace with calisthenics and West Point rigid steps (legs kept straight as possible).

Session 2: Distance 1⅝ miles.
> Walk ⅝ of a mile briskly, alternate slow, medium and brisk walking with a slow trot and West Point stance exercise (erect, but not rigid posture).

Session 3: Distance 1⅝ miles.
> Walk ¾ of a mile briskly with the same variations as in Session 2, week 7.

Week 8

Session 1: Distance 1¾ miles.
> Walking briskly ⅞ of a mile with variations of a slow, medium walk, calisthenics, West Point stance and trotting.

Session 2: Distance 1¾ miles.
> Walking briskly 1 mile with variations of slow, medium walk, calisthenics, West Point stance and trotting.

Session 3: Distance 1¾ miles.
> Same instructions as in Session 2, week 8.

Week 9

Session 1: Distance 1⅞ miles.
> Brisk walk 1⅛ miles with variations of slow, medium walk, calisthenics, West Point stance and trotting.

Session 2: Distance 1⅞ miles.
> Brisk walk 1¼ miles with variations of slow, medium walk, calisthenics, West Point stance and trotting.

Session 3: Distance 1⅞ miles.
> Same instructions as in Session 2, week 9.

WEEK 10

Session 1: Distance 1⅜ miles.
> Brisk walk with variations of slow, medium walk, calisthenics, West Point stance and trotting.

Session 2: Distance 1½ miles.
> Same instructions as in Session 1, week 10.

Session 3: Distance 1½ miles.
> Same instructions as in Session 1, week 10.

WEEK 11

Session 1: Distance 1⅝ miles.
> Brisk walk with variations of slow, medium walk, calisthenics, West Point stance and trotting.

Session 2: Distance 1¾ miles.
> Same instructions as in Session 1, week 11.

Session 3: Distance 2 miles.
> Same instructions as in Session 1, week 11.

WEEK 12

Session 1: Distance 2 miles.
> Brisk walk.

Session 2: Distance 2⅛ miles.
> Again, brisk walk for ¼ of a mile, moderate walk ¼ of a mile, trot for ¼ of a mile, West Point stance for ⅛ of a mile, brisk walk ¾ of a mile, moderate walk with calisthenics for ½ of a mile.

Session 3: Distance 2¼ miles.
> Graduation Ceremony. Brisk walk for 2¼ miles.

CHAPTER 5

Strength Development

What does strength mean to the weekend athlete—or, in fact, to the serious competitive athlete? First of all, it is a component of fitness. If we are going to engage in a sport, we need a certain amount of strength and muscular endurance. Further than that, it feels good to be strong. Physical strength allows us to move easily, to perform our daily tasks easily, engage in our sport with pleasure, and it gives us confidence that we control our bodies—not the other way around.

Since most of us are not wrestlers or shot putters, strength means—more than anything else—how well, how energetically we move our own bodies. A strong arm, strong abdominal muscles, a strong back and powerful legs can mean a sizzling, dynamite serve in tennis or a harrowing spike in volleyball. Strength is simply a factor—not the only factor—in how well we wield the implements of sport. Any tennis pro who has crossed rackets with Jimmy Connors or Billie Jean King on the pro-tennis circuit has little doubt that these athletes are strong. The big hitters on the pro-golf tour are strong. Jack Nicklaus, Tom Weiskopf and Johnny Miller are strong and they all have conditioning programs to develop that important component of their games. Baseball superstars Johnny Bench, Reggie Jackson and Dave Kingman are strong and they work at being strong.

In terms of our sports activities, I believe we can present a meaningful definition of strength and what it does for us: *Strength is the quality that allows us to move our bodies and/or the implements of our sport in a powerful, effective manner for a sustained period of time.*

The best base for a strength-development program is one that strengthens the entire body symmetrically. If we can accept the premise that a body that is strong all over feels better, functions better and plays tennis or skis better, then a total-fitness approach makes more sense than concentrating only on tennis or skiing muscles. In the chapters dealing with the various sports, I will recommend special exercises for each sport or sports category. But our basic strength and muscular-endurance program will benefit the entire body, regardless of the sports application.

If You Don't Use It, You'll Lose It

There's another factor concerning physical strength and muscular endurance that must be understood: they are continually trying to slip away. In order to increase strength, we must regularly apply graduated overloads to muscle tissue. In order to maintain strength and develop muscular endurance at a particular level, we must regularly apply a constant workload for protracted periods of time. As soon as we stop doing these things, a muscle starts going down hill. It doesn't take long for that muscle to become flacid and flabby. There's an old saying among fitness people: "If you don't use it, you'll lose it."

A Calisthenics and Weight-Training Program

The best all-around strength-development program I've come across for people who are involved in a sport and wish to improve bodily performance was designed to upgrade the physical capabilities of fire fighters. The program was developed by Richard O. Keelor, Ph.D., director of program development for the President's Council on Physical Fitness and Sports. "Just like athletes," remarked Dr. Keelor, "fire fighters perform a great variety of physical activities. They pull, they carry, they climb, they lift, they crawl and they run. They've got to be able to do it all, so they must be conditioned to do all these things."

The program combines calisthenics and weight training. The calisthenics are suitable for both men and women. In fact, even the weight program can be used by women, since it does not specify the amount of weight to be employed in the exercises. Women may prefer the alternative weight-training program I have provided later in this chapter which was designed for females and was printed in the January, 1975, issue of *WomenSports* Magazine. Since many people have misconceptions about weight training, it should be made clear that I am not talking about "body building." The body builders use weights to develop muscles for appearance, not for functional application. Second, weight training will not make you muscle-bound; it will make you stronger. Third, women needn't fear that weight training will give them big muscles. It won't—women don't have the hormones that cause bulky muscle mass in men. Today, all of the top female athletes are using weight-training techniques. Most agree that they are not only stronger, but have improved figures and body dimensions.

Here is Dr. Keelor's advice to the reader who wishes to begin this strength program:

> This program is designed to tone up large skeletal muscles and improve strength. While this is a balanced strength program, it is not a body building course. Therefore, we don't recommend lifting heavy weights, but rather, lifting a moderate weight with which you can do the suggested number of repetitions. It would be much better to increase the number of repetitions for a particular exercise than to lift a very heavy weight. If, however, you are lifting a weight which you know to be near your limit, someone should always be on hand to help you with your lift, if you need it.

In strength work, we use the terms "sets" and "repetitions." *Repetitions* are the number of times we execute a single exercise. Normally, eight repetitions = one set.

You will note that Dr. Keelor has not specified the amount of weight to be used in the exercise program. There's a good reason for this. If weights are specified, inevitably you'll find people trying to do more than they are physically prepared to do. Instead, we are going to ask you to invest one exercise session in finding out how much weight you should be using for each exercise. Here's a way to do that. Experiment with each lift until you find a weight that you can handle easily for the minimum number of repetitions and the minimum number of sets. This is your first week's workout. Gradually increase reps and sets until you reach the maximum number recommended. Then add a little more weight (3–5 pounds) and go back to the minimum number of reps and sets again. You can continue advancing in this manner until you find difficulty in lifting any more weight. From there on, increase reps and sets only.

1. Half Squats

Assume comfortable erect stance, feet shoulder width apart, hands on hips:
(1) While inhaling, slowly lower buttocks by bending knees until tops of legs are parallel to floor.
(2) Return to the starting position while exhaling.
DO NOT DO A FULL SQUAT.
Sets and Reps: 2–3 sets, 10–20 reps.
Note: Discontinue this exercise and advance to exercise 9 when you can do the recommended reps and sets for 3 or 4 weeks.

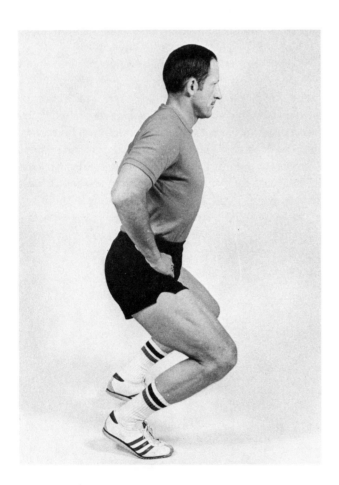

2. Calf Raise

Stand erect, hands on hips, feet spread 6–12 inches:
(1) Raise body up on toes, lifting heels.
(2) Return to starting position. Breathe normally.
Sets and Reps: 2–3 sets, 15–20 reps.
Note: Discontinue this exercise and advance to exercise 10 when you can do the recommended reps and sets for 3 or 4 weeks.

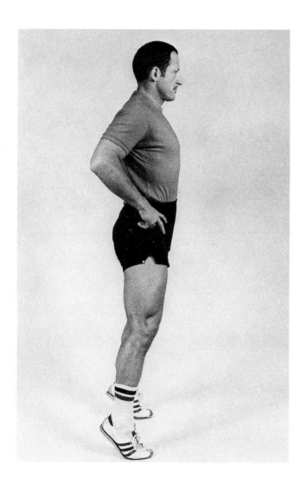

3. Pushups

Lie prone, hands outside shoulders, fingers pointed forward, weight on balls of feet:
(1) Straighten arms, keeping back, hips and knees straight.
(2) Slowly return to starting position.
Sets and Reps: 2–3 sets, 10–20 reps.

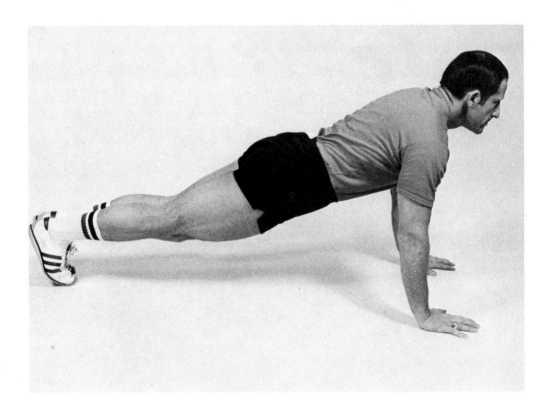

4. Modified Situps

Lie on back, legs bent, arms at side:
(1) While exhaling, curl head and shoulders off floor.
(2) Slowly return to starting position inhaling in the process.
Sets and Reps: 1–2 sets, 15–20 reps.
Note: When you can meet the specified reps and sets, try the exercise with hands locked behind the head and work up to the same reps and sets. Continue for 3 or 4 weeks, then advance to exercise 19.

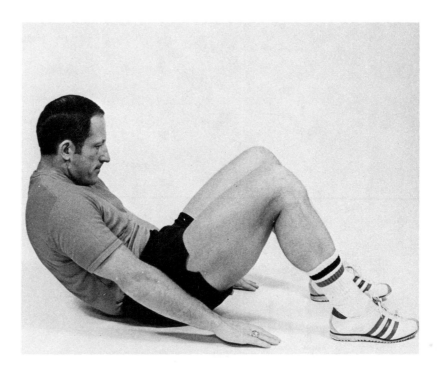

5. Alternate Dumbbell Press

Assume comfortable seated position on a flat bench. Hold dumbbells with an overhand grip at shoulder height:
(1) Fully extend right arm over head.
(2) Lower right arm and simultaneously extend left arm.
Sets and Reps: 2–3 sets, 10–15 reps each arm.
Note: You can advance to a heavier dumbbell after you have done maximum reps and sets for 3 or 4 weeks.

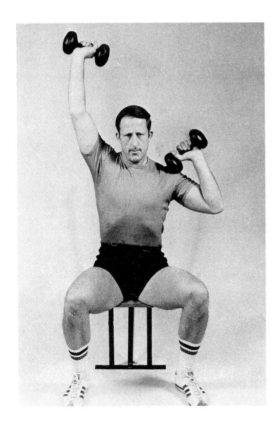

6. Military Press

Take a wide overhand grasp of bar, wide foot stance and bring bar to chest position:
(1) Exhaling, slowly extend bar overhead until arms are completely extended.
(2) Inhaling, slowly return bar to starting position until it touches chest.
Sets and Reps: 2–3 sets, 8–12 reps.
Note: When you reach specified reps and sets, add a little weight. Continue for 3–4 weeks then advance to exercise 12.

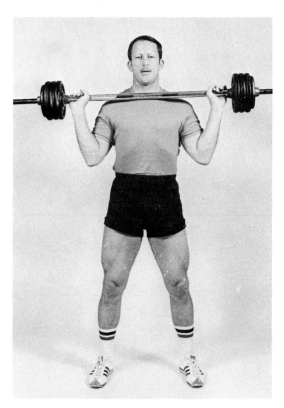
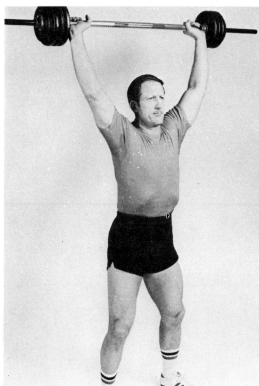

7. Lightweight Dead Lifts with Shrug

Assume wide foot stance, lower buttocks and bend knees until bar can be reached with extended arms. Take a wide reverse grip (one hand overhand, one underhand):
(1) While exhaling, lift first with legs until bar reaches knees, then straighten knees and back simultaneously until you reach an upright position.
(2) While in upright position, shrug shoulders up and backward.
(3) Return bar to starting position, inhaling. Use legs to lower bar as in lifting.
Sets and Reps: 2–3 sets, 8–12 reps.
USE ONLY LIGHT WEIGHT.

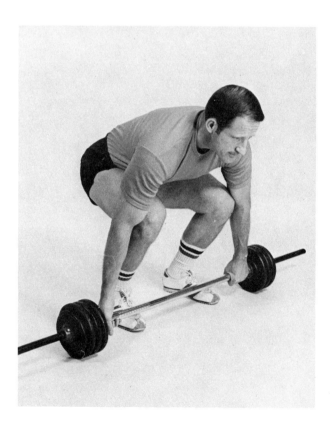

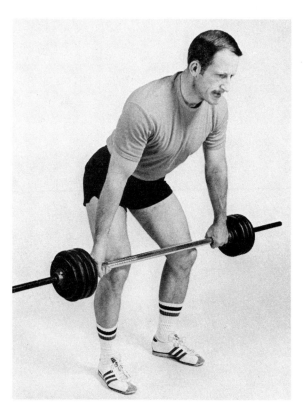 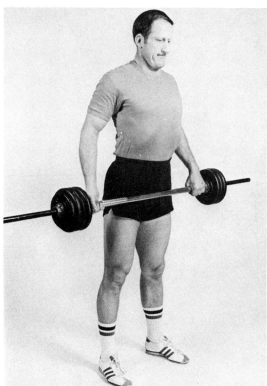

8. Seated Alternate Dumbbell Curls

Assume a comfortable seated position on a flat bench. Hold dumbbells with an underhand grip (so palms face up) arms fully extended at side:
(1) Slowly raise left arm, bending only the elbow until arm is fully flexed.
(2) Slowly lower left arm and simultaneously begin raising right arm to its fully flexed position. Breathe normally.
Sets and Reps: 2–3 sets, 8–10 reps on each arm.

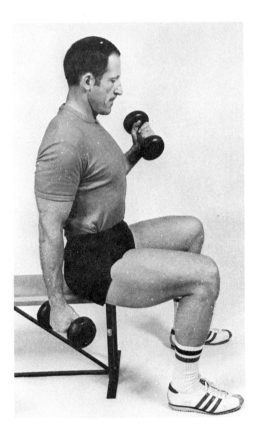
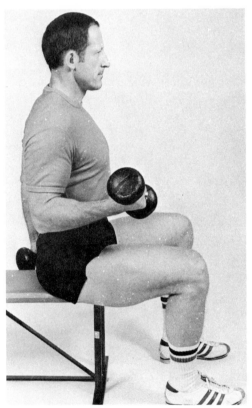

9. Half Squats with Barbell

Take a wide overhand grip on bar and lift it overhead, resting it comfortably behind neck. Assume a comfortable standing position with feet shoulder width apart (2 x 4 board under heels may be used for balance):

(1) Inhaling, slowly lower body by bending knees until tops of legs are parallel to floor or buttocks rest on a 12-inch bench.

(2) Exhaling, raise body upward by extending knees until body is fully upright.

DO NOT LOWER TO A FULL SQUAT POSITION. USE LIGHT WEIGHT.

Sets and Reps: 2–3 sets, 12–15 reps.

Note: This exercise replaces exercise 1.

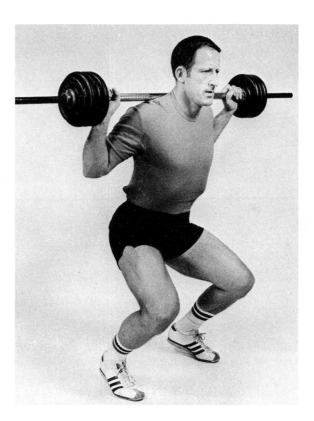

10. Calf Raise with Barbell

Take a wide underhand grip on bar and lift it overhead, resting it comfortably behind neck. Assume shoulder-width stance:

(1) Raise up on toes lifting heels as high as possible.

(2) Slowly lower heels to starting position. Breathe normally.

Note: A 2 x 4 board placed under the toes may be used for fuller range of action.

Sets and Reps: 2–3 sets, 10–15 reps.

Note: This exercise replaces exercise 2.

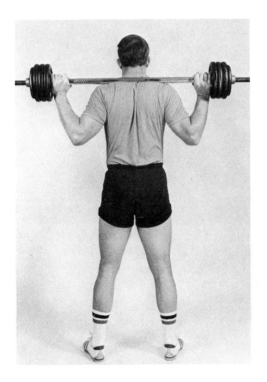
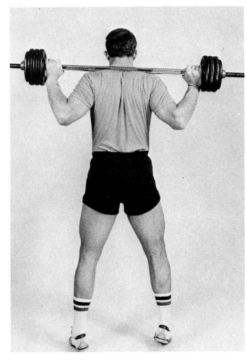

11. Dumbbell Bench Press

Start in comfortable prone position on flat bench, feet spread and securely positioned.
Hold dumbbells (turned out) at lowest comfortable position:
(1) Exhaling, push dumbbells upward slowly until arms are fully extended and
    dumbbells touch over chest.
(2) Inhaling, slowly lower dumbbells to starting position.
Sets and Reps: 2–3 sets, 8–12 reps.

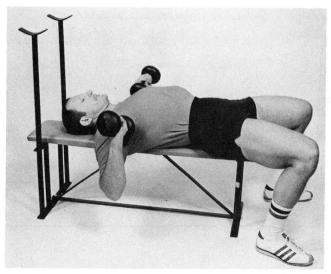

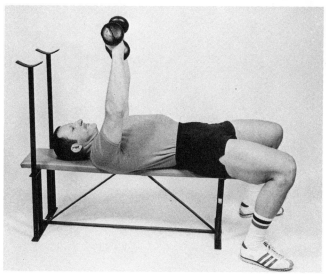

12. Barbell Clean and Press

Take a wide overhand grasp of bar, wide foot stance and lower buttocks below shoulder height:
(1) Exhaling, lift first with legs, then back, snapping bar to chest.
(2) Taking a short breath, first push weight overhead, exhaling until weight is fully extended.
(3) Return weight to chest and then to starting position inhaling on the way down.
Sets and Reps: 2–3 sets, 6–10 reps.
Note: This exercise replaces exercise 6.

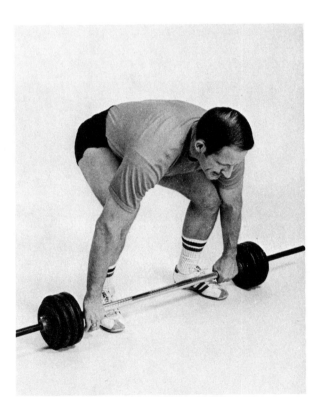

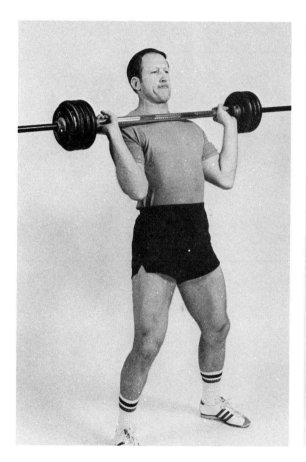
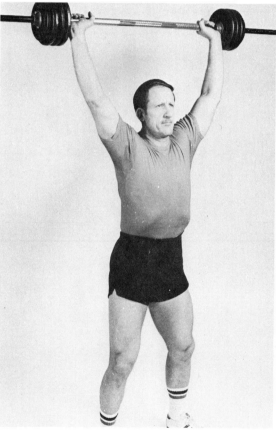

13. Barbell Bench Press

Take a comfortable prone position on a flat bench, feet spread and securely positioned. Take wide, overhand grip on bar with arms extended:
(1) Inhaling, slowly lower bar from extended position until it touches chest.
(2) Exhaling, push bar up from the chest until arms are fully extended.
Sets and Reps: 2–3 sets, 6–10 reps.
CAUTION: This exercise should not be performed with heavy weight unless someone is spotting.

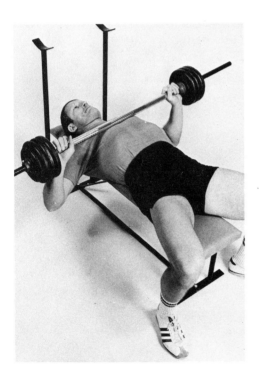 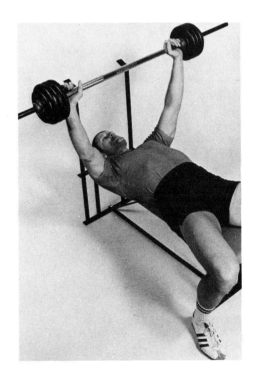

14. Upright Rows

Standing with feet spread, take a close overhand grip on bar about a thumb's distance apart. Hold bar at belt line:

(1) Raise bar up to chin level with elbows as high as possible.

(2) Slowly return bar to belt line. Breathe normally.

Sets and Reps: 2–3 sets, 10–15 reps.

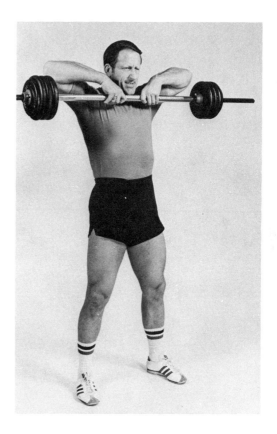

15. Bent-over Rows

Grasp the bar with a wide overhand grip several inches outside the shoulders. Bend knees and the waist about 45°:

(1) With the bar hanging almost touching the ground from extended arms, pull it up until it touches the chest.

(2) Inhaling, slowly lower it to the original position.

Sets and Reps: 2–3 sets, 8–12 reps.

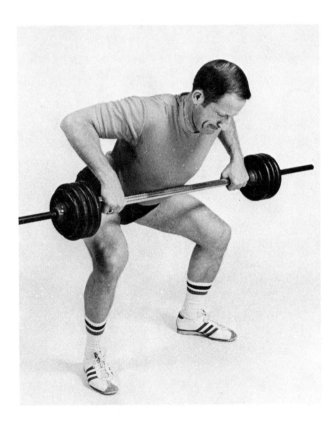

16. Barbell Curls

Take a shoulder-width underhand grip on the bar and stand erect with feet comfortably spread, arms completely extended:
(1) Exhaling slowly, bring bar upward by bending the elbows until arm is completely flexed and bar has reached shoulder level.
(2) Inhaling slowly, return the bar slowly to the starting position.
Sets and Reps: 2–3 sets, 8–12 reps.

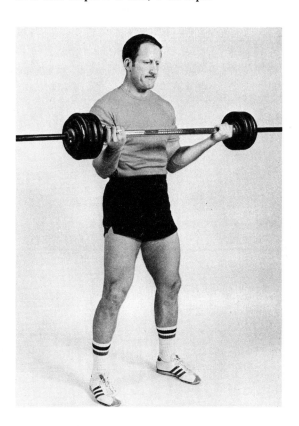

17. Seated Tricep Extensions

Take a comfortable seated position with a shoulder-width overhand grip on bar. Hold bar directly overhead.

(1) Slowly lower bar down behind head, bending only the elbows as far as comfortable. Inhale on the way down.

(2) Keeping elbows pointed straight ahead (do not allow them to point to the sides) slowly raise bar to the original position. Exhale on the way up.

Sets and Reps: 2–3 sets, 8–12 reps.

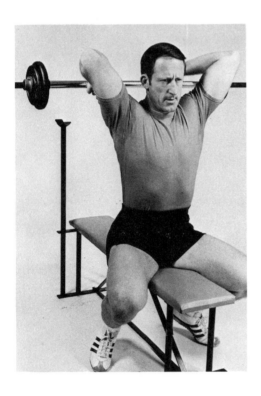 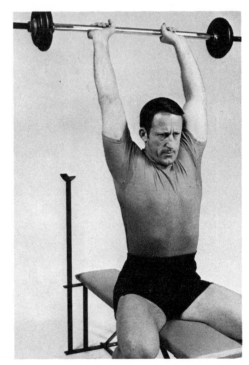

18. Leg Thrusts

Taking a wide grip, lift bar overhead until it can be rested comfortably behind neck. Assume a comfortable standing position, with feet apart.

(1) Slowly step forward with right leg, bending left knee until it touches floor.

(2) Shoving off from right leg, push back to original standing position.

(3) Repeat with left leg forward.

Sets and Reps: 2 sets, 6–10 reps on each leg.

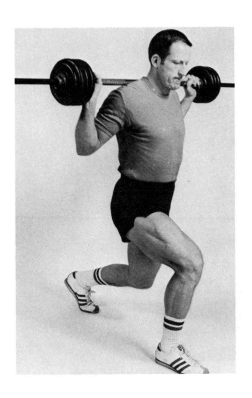 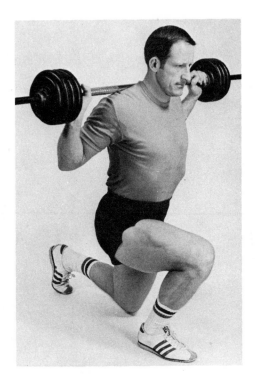

19. Situps (Slant Board)

Lie on back (preferably on slant board), knees bent, feet hooked under strap, fingers laced behind head:
(1) Curl torso to upright position, touching elbows to knees. Exhale on the way up.
(2) Return to starting position. Inhale on way down.
Note: Difficulty can be increased by touching right elbow to left knee and left elbow to right knee.
Sets and Reps: 2 sets, 20–30 reps.

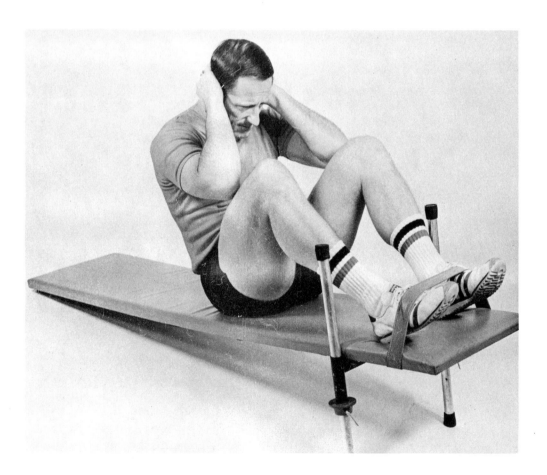

A Weight Training Program
Specially Designed for Women

The following material was excerpted from an article that appeared in *WomenSports* Magazine in January 1975. Writer Shirley Biondi interviewed exercise physiologist Jack Wilmore, who has taught physical education at several major universities. Jack has become the leading authority on weight training for women and his successes should reassure women who are concerned about acquiring "bulging muscles" as a result of a weight program.

Wilmore taught weight training to women exclusively—270 U.C. at Davis students—who met three times a week. More than two years of experiments with over 600 female weight trainers at Davis have proven that women and men can lift weights side by side—the man develops muscles, and the woman develops a strong and shapely figure. Why? Wilmore explains.

"Weight training for women has traditionally been taboo," he says. "Female athletes saw that men on a weight-training program developed huge biceps. So they said to themselves, 'Even if lifting weights would make me stronger, I'm not going to risk getting all those ugly muscles.' And so, women in the U.S. never used any systematic program of weight training."

But six years ago Dr. Harmon Brown and Wilmore studied seven nationally ranked girl and women field-event athletes, five of whom used intensive weight training, and this changed his mind about women and weights. After six months of weight training, all of the athletes increased their strength up to fifty-three percent, and their body proportions improved, but without bulging muscles.

"Large muscles in men are the result of the body's secretion of the male hormone testosterone," explains Wilmore. "Women secrete this hormone too, but in much smaller amounts. So most women can lift weights without developing bulky muscles and with quicker results than traditional exercise programs."

Wilmore began his experiment at U.C. at Davis three and a half years ago with one class and only four students. To increase enrollment, he visited body-mechanics classes and told the girls that weight training would produce better, quicker results. He managed to round up seventeen skeptical, but adventuresome, students.

To prove his theory, Wilmore took more than sixty measurements of each girl at the beginning and at the end of the ten-week course. The girls showed up to a thirty-percent increase in strength; some girls ended the class as much as eighty-percent stronger. And, even without dieting, the girls lost as much as four inches overall from waist, hips and thighs, with a slight increase in bust size.

For the potential weight trainer, Wilmore has some advice. Anyone over twenty-five, or with a history of medical problems, should see if her physician has any objections. Then if the doctor approves, since everyone's body proportions are genetically determined, Wilmore further cautions, one should not expect miracles: "If you begin the program looking like Totie Fields or Peter Ustinov, don't expect to finish up looking like Raquel Welch or Mark Spitz."

Body weight consists of lean weight (muscles, bones and organs) and fat weight. Each person's proportions of fat and lean weight are different, which may explain why your friend, with a similar body type, who weighs the same as you or even more, can look firmer than you. If you have a high proportion of lean weight, you look "solid." Without it, you look "flabby."

People who weight-train increase their lean weight and reduce their proportion of fat, says Wilmore. Some people call this "reproportioning the body."

Happily, fat weight usually comes off first from the places it is deposited heaviest, Wilmore explains. So a consistent program of weight training reduces proportions where a person wants to lose most.

When you're ready to begin, wear clothes that are comfortable and not confining. And try to store the weights in a place (preferably with a cement floor) where your exercise sessions won't be interrupted by distractions.

You should spend five to ten minutes on the warm-ups, and about thirty minutes with the weights. "Start each exercise with a weight you can lift comfortably ten consecutive times," says Wilmore. "You'll have to experiment to find the proper weight.

"Stay with this weight for several sessions, until you can lift it comfortably sixteen to eighteen times. Then, move on to the next heaviest weight.

"Lifting too little weight will mean slower results, but lifting too much can result in serious injury. And always have someone with you when you lift weights over your head!

"At first, you'll get really sore," Wilmore advises, "mainly because you're probably using muscles for the first time that you didn't even know existed. But after five or six sessions, the soreness should go away and the results begin to show. This should encourage you to stay at it.

"Strength is a very basic component of any athletic performance," Wilmore says. "We've proven that people who lift weights in a conscientious training program become stronger, firmer and even more physically attractive. So I can't see any reason not to use weight training for all athletes—male and female alike."

WILMORE'S WARM-UPS (10-15 MINUTES)

1. Situps (20 times)
   Lie on your back with your knees bent at a 45-degree angle. Put your hands behind your neck. Pull up to a sitting position, and then lower yourself to the starting position. Repeat.
2. Modified Pushups (20 times)
   Lie down on your stomach, with your arms straight out in front of your chest, touching

the floor. Lower the upper half of your body to the floor until you touch your chest to the floor, then use your arms to push yourself back up. Repeat.

3. Hops (20 times)

   Hang your arms loosely at your sides. Hop on one foot 20 times, and then the other.

4. Knee to Chest (10 times each leg)

   Stand up straight. Pull your right knee up to your chest while standing on your left leg. Use your arms to pull the knee into the chest. Return your leg to the floor and repeat with your right leg.

5. Trunk Circles (20 times)

   Stand with your feet shoulder-width apart and your hands on your hips. Bending at the waist, slowly rotate your upper body forward, to the right, to the left, and then return to the forward position. Slowly bend closer to the floor with each repetition.

WILMORE'S WEIGHT LIFTS

Barbells

Begin with a weight you can handle easily. Refer to previous weight program for progression of reps and sets. ALWAYS HAVE SOMEONE WITH YOU WHEN YOU LIFT WEIGHTS OVER YOUR HEAD!

1. Standing Press

   Stand with your feet shoulder-width apart. Bend your knees halfway. Reach down and grab the bar with your palms facing the floor, hands spread about shoulder-width apart. Lift the weight to the starting position by straightening your legs. As the bar approaches your hips, bend your legs again, allowing you to snap your elbows under the bar. Keep your back straight. From the standing position, with the bar at chest level, lift the weight straight up and over your head, locking the elbows out straight. Return the weight to starting position. Repeat.

2. Two-arm Curl

   Standing up, pick up the bar with your palms toward the ceiling. Bring the bar to a position to rest against your thighs, with your arms straight down, while you are in a standing position, feet spread shoulder-width apart. Using only your arms, raise the bar until it touches your chest and then lower it to the thigh, fully extending the elbows. Repeat.

3. Bent Rowing

   Bend your knees halfway and bend forward at the waist. With your back parallel to the floor, grasp the bar with palms toward the floor, hands shoulder-width apart. Using the arms only, lift the barbell to the chest and return it to the floor. Repeat.

4. Half-squat

   Stand with your feet shoulder-width apart. Bend your arms, with your hands near your shoulder, palms toward the ceiling. Have your partner place the barbell on your hands, on top of your shoulders, behind your neck. With your back straight, lower the weight by bending the knees halfway (as if you're sitting down) and return to the standing position. Repeat.

5. Bench Press

Lie down on your back on a bench with your knees bent halfway, feet flat on the bench. Have your partner hand you the barbell with your arms straight above your chest, shoulder-width apart. Lower the weight until it touches your chest and then straighten your arms again. Repeat.

Dumbbell Exercises

1. Flying Motion (suggested starting weight: 5–10 pounds)

   Lie on your back on a bench. With a dumbbell in each hand, straighten your arms out to the side with a slight bend in the elbow. Bring the weights overhead, crossing your arms, and return to the side position. Repeat.

2. Lateral Raise (suggested starting weight: 5–10 pounds)

   Stand with your feet comfortably apart, with a dumbbell in each hand and your arms at your sides. Raise the arms up sideways (as if you're flying), to bring your arms to an overhead position, with the two weights touching. Return to your side. Repeat.

3. Side Bend (suggested starting weight: 5–10 pounds)

   Stand with feet comfortably apart. With a dumbbell in the left hand, slowly bend at the waist to the right, then return to the upright position. Repeat several times, then transfer dumbbell to the right, and repeat exercise by bending to the left.

CHAPTER 6

Golf Exercises

The electric golf car has taken the exercise value out of a round of golf—not that it really had very much to begin with. Anyone who feels that he is getting a workout from eighteen holes of golf needs help. There are golfers who walk the course and carry their clubs. This certainly has fitness benefits, if it is part of a comprehensive fitness program.

The best way to present exercise to the golfer is to show him how strength, flexibility and endurance will make his weekly game of golf a lot more fun and even lower his handicap. This is a realistic promise and I'll tell you why. What usually happens when you are in a golfing situation that calls for a little extra distance off the tee or the fairway? Let me guess. You let it all out! You swing the club harder—but you don't hit the ball harder. You end up off-balance, watching the ball slicing eagerly toward the woods.

Suppose you took your regular golf swing, added a bit more suppleness to your hip and shoulder turn, injected a little more strength into the back and shoulder muscles, put a bit of the iron into the forearms, wrists and fingers? Do you think that you could get that additional twenty or thirty yards? Probably a lot more. Every golfer on the pro tour knows this and they all have regular exercise and conditioning programs to get as much as possible out of the physical equipment that they have. Gary Player was one of the first of the leading golfers to demonstrate that a program of strength and endurance development could turn a good golfer into a great one.

Laura Baugh, one of the brighter lights of the Ladies PGA, tells us how golfers should regard their physical conditioning:

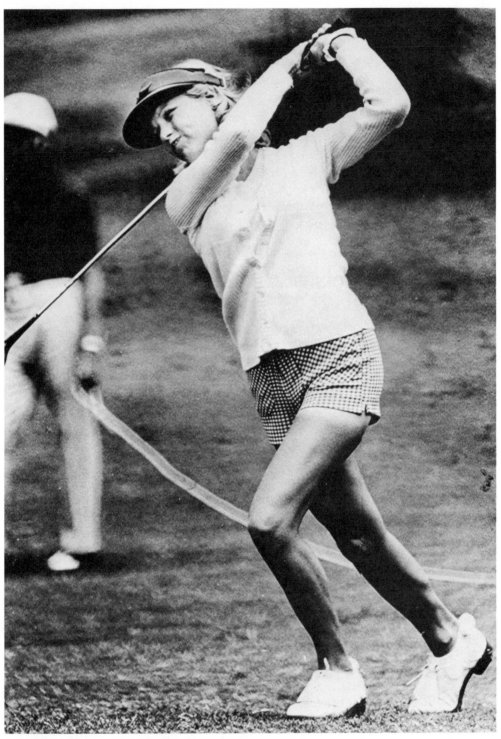

Laura Baugh is one of many professional golfers who consider fitness an important part of preparation for competition. (UPI)

Many people think of golfers as not being really the physical fitness types . . . maybe a little overweight and a little out of shape. Well, this is sometimes true. At least, it was in the past more than it is now.

There are many things about our life-styles that make it difficult to stay in shape. There are flights and the waiting at airports when you have nothing to do for several hours, except maybe eat something or drink something. Then there are the cocktail parties and luncheons and receptions at the clubs.

So you really have to bear down to stay in shape. Today, most of the women on the tour—just like the men—are in shape. Even the weekend golfer will play much better golf if he or she is in good physical condition. You need endurance to get around that golf course for several hours, especially in hot weather; and you want your mind to be alert if you're playing a match, which will not be the case, if you're fatigued.

A golfer should try to make regular exercise a part of the daily routine, whether it's walking or jogging. It's got to become part of your routine so that it becomes part of you. When I'm off the tour, I run every day. When I'm out on the tour, it's difficult to find the time or a place to run, so I travel with a jumping rope.

I have one additional word of advice for the weekend golfer. Golfers should warm up before a round of golf just as other athletes do before their sport. This is very important. Some stretching and flexibility exercises are recommended. And part of your warm-up should be hitting golf balls for ten minutes or so. This will get your golf muscles loose and ready for what they are going to be required to do.

Flexibility for Golfers

I would advise a golfer who can to embark on a total fitness program including the strength, endurance and flexibility components outlined elsewhere in this book. Such an approach would have dramatic results for the average weekend golfer. But if there is any one thing that can help the average golf swing, it is flexibility.

Golfers want to get that clubhead back. They want to get the extension on the backswing and in the follow-through that provides controlled power. Here are some flexibility exercises that will help your golf swing:

1. Do a brief warm-up routine such as that described in the "Warm-up Flexibility" chapter. Then do the first four flexibility exercises. These are all beneficial in developing suppleness in the torso.
2. A variation on exercise 4 (trunk twister) in the "Warm-up" chapter is to place a golf club across your back—held in place by your elbows—and rotate your shoulders from side to side.

3. A further variation of this exercise that promotes a full body turn is executed by locking the hands behind the head, with elbows extended. Then, alternately, bend and twist touching the right elbow to the left knee—left elbow to right knee.

4. An easy-to-perform, yet quite useful, exercise is the parallel arm swing. Here's how to do it:

Starting position: Stand erect, feet shoulder-width apart and hands hanging slightly in front of the body.

Action:
   (1) Swing both arms to the right and upward as far as possible, rotating the hips in a smooth motion.
   (2) Swing both arms down in front of the body and to the left as far as possible.

Suggested repetitions: 10-15.

Note: You will immediately feel how this action duplicates the basic moves of the golf swing and stretches the golf muscles.

Put Power in Your Hands, Wrists and Forearms

Here's some good advice by New York Yankees outfielder, Roy White, on how to build up the hands, wrists and forearms. These parts of the body establish the mechanical link between the golf club (or baseball bat) and the rest of the body. They can either be a weak link or contribute their share of power. Roy says:

> There are many ways to build strong hands, wrists and forearms. You can start by constantly squeezing a hard rubber ball, first with your right hand and then with your left hand. Wrist curls with dumbbells will build strong forearms and wrists; be sure to do both forward and reverse curls, so that you avoid overdeveloping one set of arm muscles.
> Another exercise involves rolling a weight onto a broomstick. Fasten a fifteen-pound weight to the end of a rope and tie the other end of the rope to the center of a fifteen-inch broomstick. Extend your arms to the front parallel to the ground and slowly roll the weight up and down, winding the rope around the broomstick as you rotate your wrists. I begin this exercise with three sets of five repetitions, and work up from there.

Golfers can use Roy's exercises during the winter together with the complete off-season program developed by Gary Wiren, director of golf instruction and education for the PGA of America, an expert on all aspects of physical fitness and recognized authority on the golf swing. The following is reprinted with the permission of *Golf Digest* Magazine:

In football, basketball, baseball, track, swimming, wrestling, gymnastics and other sports, there are off-season drills and exercises designed to produce improved performance. Since golf has varying degrees of the physical requirements of other sports, why not train for golf? If your mind already is thinking about next season, how about getting your body ready as well? Wouldn't it be a delight to open the season and not have your clubs feel like strangers and your body feel as though it had never played the game?

You don't have to take a winter vacation to the sun to prepare yourself. The office, front room or basement can be a great training ground.

Club professional Bob Ellsworth of Hood River, Ore., never before a tournament winner in his section, came out of a snow-filled winter a few years ago to win the Section PGA and Northwest Open early in the spring. His entire practice that off-season had been indoors, where he worked on an indoor swing training and improvement program. Debbie Massey, recent qualifying medalist in the U.S. Women's Amateur, keeps her game sharp during the winter by hitting balls into a net at Stowe, Vt., where she teaches skiing.

Endurance is not a particularly critical element in the striking of a golf ball once or twice, or even 10 times. But, when you have been walking for more than three hours, possibly even carrying or pulling your clubs, and you need to hit a crucial shot, endurance becomes important. A fatigued body just does not produce fine motor skills as precisely as a body that is fresh. Ask yourself, "How do I perform on the last few holes of the round?" If the answer is, "Not very well," then I prescribe regular running or bicycle riding during the off-season to build up endurance to carry you through a round.

Exercises or drills fall generally into two categories, those dealing with technique and those dealing with physical conditioning. The exercises I am demonstrating for you on these pages are designed to improve both your technique and the condition of the muscles that will be used in playing golf.

Use a door jamb to fix your swing center

Place your head lightly against a door jamb and, without using a club, make a full backswing and follow-through. Keep your head in contact with the jamb, allowing the head to turn to the target on the finish. By keeping your head "back" you can feel the stretch as your lower body unwinds toward the target and your back arches. This is a fine drill for learning the feeling of a fixed center in the swing.

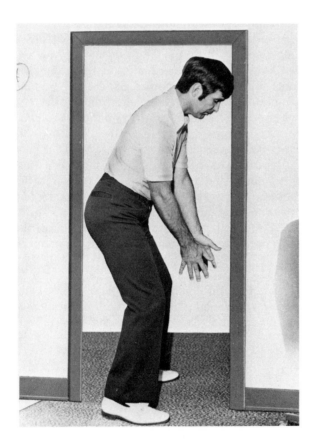

Turn and tug to get hands high

This exercise increases your ability to make a big turn and get your hands high. If you used only your left arm, the length of your backswing would be abbreviated. By placing the fingers of your right hand on the shaft and firmly tugging, you will stretch further and thereby increase your flexibility and turn. Keep your left arm extended and wrist flat to get the greatest feeling of stretch. A similar effect can be gained from swinging with a 20-to-26-ounce driver, allowing the extra weight to carry you beyond your normal stretched position. Your regular driver can be weighted artificially with such devices as lead tape and heavy head covers.

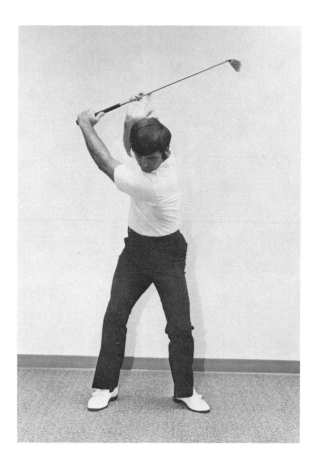

Swing with left side to feel release

If you have had trouble feeling a release in your swing, grip your left forearm just above the wrist and make a swing with your left side and the right hand going along for support. When you get near the hitting area, you'll realize the tremendous power centrifugal force provides without your having to interject leverage action with the hands.

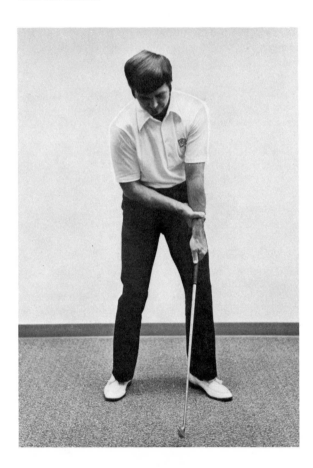

Preset the hands to develop late hit

Starting with your left arm straight and your left wrist flat, set the clubhead at about 110 degrees from the vertical and tuck your right elbow toward your tummy. Now, with the knees flexed and the body tilted forward, make a big shoulder turn, drive with your legs and pull with your left arm toward your target. Let the release of energy happen by itself. By presetting your hands in the air and starting from this position, you take away much of the tendency to strike early. Centrifugal force is realized much more easily. Use this drill when you're plagued by hitting from the top and when you want to get the feeling of "swing" rather than "hit." Place a target line on the ground, if you want to work on direction as well.

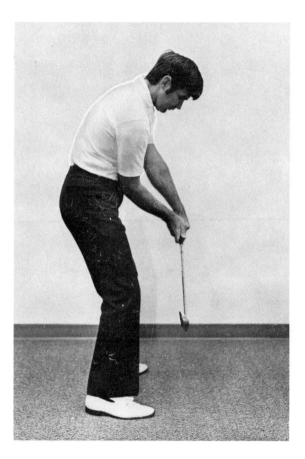

Point the handle to stay on plane

Grip the club in the middle of the shaft, make a backswing, then start into your forward swing. Midway through, check to see that the handle end of the club points toward your flight line. Your swing by choice may be flat or upright, but, to be in plane, a line drawn through the shaft and extending out the butt end of the club must point to the flight line.

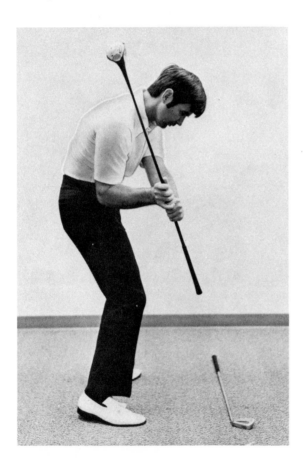

Extend firm left arm and hold it to correct collapsing

This drill requires that you hold the pictured static position: (1) weight to the left, (2) left arm nearly at chest height, fully extended and rotated 180 degrees from its position in the downswing, (3) right hand crossed over and lightly on top, (4) head well back. Hold that position for 10 seconds, go halfway into your backswing and return to the extended position and hold again. The muscle memory drill works wonders for a collapsing left arm. If you tend to slice, make the clubface point to the ground when you reach this position.

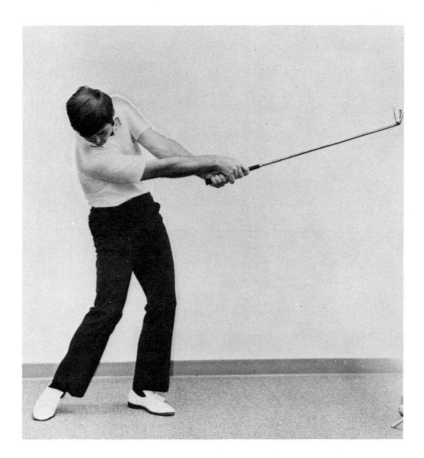

Club hitting surface after impact to develop later release

Practice making swings which reach the bottom of their arc slightly after contacting the ball. On the turf, you will get grass after you hit the ball, but indoors you simply will hit a mark on the target side of the ball. This will be a great aid in helping you develop a later, timed release and produce greater clubhead speed.

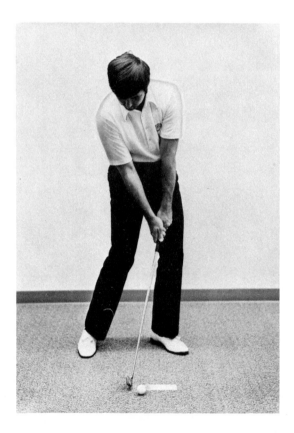

Stretch to more distance

This is one position in a simple yoga routine called Salute to the Sun. (The complete routine can be found in most elementary yoga books.) Flexibility or stretching exercises should be a part of any golf shape-up program. Lack of flexibility is one of the chief causes of loss of distance.

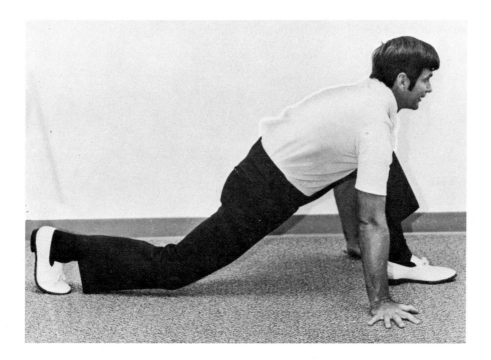

Firm the flexors to hit ball further

You have some magic muscles for golf in your left arm. They are the flexors, the grasping muscles in your forearms. Firm flexors allow you to strike the ball without the grip turning in your hands. Practice this exercise while sitting in a chair. Extend your left arm and grip a club in your left hand, using only the last three fingers. Rotate the club from an open to closed position. Then, flex and relax your grip. A winter of this exercise in front of the TV or at your desk during phone calls can dramatically improve your grip and distance.

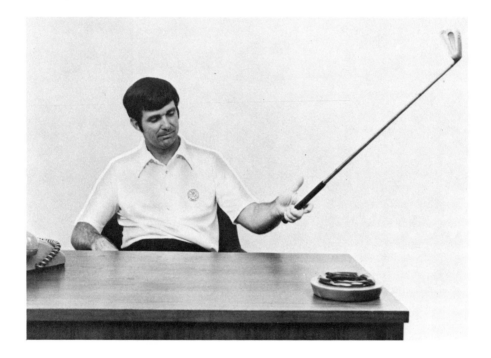

CHAPTER 7

Exercises for Tennis, Racket Sports, Handball

Tennis and other racket sports present a number of training and conditioning challenges to the weekend player. Tennis today is a very popular recreational activity. Because it has taken on some degree of social or status appeal, many people who play, or play at, tennis are not athletic. They are not conditioned for the kinds of things they may end up trying to do. Even the serious tennis player who is aware of his or her physical limitations may believe that these limitations are going to disappear as skill improves. Unless that person is playing tennis for several hours a day—every day—that isn't going to happen. There's no substitute for a regular conditioning program. It is significant that the world's leading tennis players—people who do play every day—all have conditioning programs.

Billie Jean King, whose list of championships is as impressive as her overhead smash, has this to say about conditioning for tennis:

Fitness and conditioning become increasingly important to the tennis player as skill improves. This is because, in order to make the shot, you've got to be able to get to the ball. Two elements of conditioning come into play here: endurance and agility. Both of these components of fitness can be improved upon. This improvement calls for a physical training program. A program that enables a player to keep his or her game strong right up to the last point of a match...even on a hot, humid day. You've got to build endurance with a running program and regularly perform the drills that improve speed, agility and footwork.

Add Speed and Agility to Your Game

You can build speed and increased agility into your tennis game by adding some variety to your jogging-running program. Racket sports call for more than straight-ahead speed. These sports require you to move forward, backward, laterally and diagonally. In order to increase your balance and agility and build speed and quickness, add these variations to your running activities. At frequent intervals, try short sprints; then slow down to a jog until you recover your wind. Try running backward, skipping sideways and in a zigzag configuration, changing direction sharply by planting one foot and pushing off in the opposite direction. Introduce hopping and skipping steps into your running; make complete turns in both directions. And any time when the weather makes running impossible, do some rope skipping.

Special Conditioning Exercises for Racket Sports

The following exercise program was developed by physical therapist Joseph Zohar. Mr. Zohar is establishing a far-reaching reputation for his work with injured athletes, but his expertise is not limited to injury-related therapy. He would rather that athletes, especially weekend athletes, invest in sufficient conditioning to prevent unnecessary strains and muscle tears. With that end in view, Mr. Zohar researched and developed a comprehensive conditioning program designed to strengthen and stretch the areas most vulnerable to injury in racket sports. He has generously provided this material for readers of this book. His complete program, which is well worth exploring by serious tennis players, can be found in his book, *Scientific Conditioning Program for Tennis*.

A Total Fitness Prescription for Racket Sports

Tennis is exhausting to the player with poor endurance. Even if you can move pretty well and make the shots, you've got to be able to play your game without undue cardio-vascular stress. Then there are players who can run the courts all day, but they're pussycats because they can't put the shot away. No power in the arms or upper body. There are weekend tennis players who can last, who have the power to return a shot—if they can reach the ball. But they have little mobility, can neither move nor stretch.

There's no reason to envy the player who can do all of these things, while you are trying to enjoy a restricted, limited game. If you belong on the tennis court at all, you should be able to hang in there with your opponent or outlast him. You should know the satisfaction of delivering an unreturnable overhand smash and the pleasure of movement without strain or pain.

Endurance Comes First

For the beginning or intermediate tennis player, cardio-vascular endurance is the first prerequisite. Don't tax yourself once or twice a week with an hour of tennis that has you running a tightrope between a bunch of missed shots on one side and a coronary arrest on the other. The game of tennis should be fun. It should satisfy some of your competitive urges and leave you feeling physically elevated—not totally spent. More advanced players should be able to reach back for a little extra stamina, even after a few hours of summer tennis. The way to do this is the way Billie Jean King and Jimmy Connors do it: build your circulatory-respiratory storehouse through a regular jogging or running program. Try the programs in the "Endurance" chapter of this book. Once you've progressed through a few weeks of regular running, your tennis game will be a piece of cake.

STRENGTH FOR TENNIS

Later in this chapter I have included a series of exercises developed by a well-known sports physical therapist that will help you to strengthen your tennis muscles in the arm, shoulder and upper body. As a base, do the exercises described in the "Strength Development" chapter. In that chapter you'll find most of the exercises that tennis coaches agree tennis players need for a power game. At the same time, you will be strengthening your entire body. There are a couple of routines you may wish to add, such as double-leg raises for the hip flexor muscles. This is another exercise that helps provide power to the service and all overhead shots:

Starting position: Lie on the back with hands clasped behind the head.
Action:
(1) Raise both legs off the floor and bring to vertical position.

(2) Slowly lower legs to the floor.
Suggested repetitions: 2–3 sets, 10–20 reps.

Try doing racket jumps to strengthen the legs. This is a good agility exercise as well. You'll see this exercise illustrated in the "Ski" section of chapter eight, where Suzy Chaffee demonstrates "bench jumping" as an advanced exercise for skiers. Racket jumping is a lot easier; you should be able to do it.

Starting position: Place your racket on the ground and stand alongside it.
Action:
(1) Jump over your racket sideways, landing softly with your knees flexed.
(2) Jump back to starting position.
(3) Repeat jumping from one side of your racket to the other.
Suggested repetitions: 2–3 sets of 10 reps.

Another exercise that is very popular among tennis players is the "Kangaroo Hop." This exercise is a tough one and you're going to have to be in pretty good shape to do it. It's great for developing leg strength and abdominal stamina. It's another of the special group of exercises that also promotes agility and "quick legs."

Starting position: Stand erect with feet together.
Action:
Leap upward, attempting to bring knees up to chest.
Suggested reps: 2–3 sets of ten reps, done as quickly as you can do them.

Warm-ups and Flexibility for Tennis and Racket Sports

Off-Court Warm-ups

Begin each regular conditioning session with the warm-up and flexibility drills described in the chapter dealing with these subjects.

On-Court Warm-ups

Prior to a round of tennis, it is important to get your muscles loose and your body temperature and respiration up a bit. The best way to do this is to begin with a slow jog around the courts for about two minutes. Then do some warm-ups for the upper body. We have suggested the simulated swimming motions as a good basic warm-up technique and it works very well for tennis. Also do the first four flexibility exercises listed in the "Warm-up and Flexibility" chapter.

Complete your warm-up by simulating your tennis strokes and various moves using your racket with the racket cover on for added resistance. Run forward toward the net, run backward toward the baseline, skip sideways, move diagonally—at the same time, move your racket through your forehand, backhand and overhead strokes. Develop your own series of moves and strokes so that you can systematically repeat this warm-up drill each time you prepare to play.

Joseph Zohar's Weight Program—General Instructions

WEIGHTS

The weights should be increased gradually and with caution, even if the exercises seem too easy at first. A common misconception is that "an exercise does not do you any good unless you really feel it." Nothing is further from the truth. The weight should not be increased until the exercise can be repeated ten times with relative ease. Do not increase if you feel undue strain or pain either during or after the exercise. When in doubt, continue to use the same weight rather than risk muscle strain, which may force discontinuing the exercise until the strain subsides. However, do not "coast" at one weight level; when ready, move up!

MAXIMUM AND OPTIMUM WEIGHTS

How much weight is the final goal? To prevent injuries such as tennis elbow and shoulder tendonitis, muscles must be strengthened to maximum levels so they can withstand strains far above the normal requirements of the game. When you are unable to increase a given weight after five consecutive sessions, it can be safely assumed that the muscles have reached maximum strength.

However, to improve playing ability, it is not necessary to strengthen the muscles to maximum level, only to optimum level. For each exercise, high and low figures indicate the optimum weight levels for men, women, boys and girls. The figures are only intended to serve as guidelines. For some persons, it may be both easy and desirable to increase the weight beyond the high figure; others may find even the low figure beyond their capacity.

When optimum weight has been reached, you have several options. You may continue to exercise with the optimum weight to maintain and reinforce your strength, increase the number of repetitions to improve muscle endurance or start a new exercise.

REPETITIONS AND ENDURANCE

Initially, each exercise should be repeated ten times, with a three- to six-second rest between lifts. After optimum weight is reached, endurance can be increased by using the same weight while gradually increasing the repetitions to twenty or even thirty. Preferably two, but no more than five repetitions can be added each session.

Relaxation

The ability to keep muscles relaxed is essential for developing a smooth tennis stroke. The three- to six-second rest between lifts helps you feel the difference between a relaxed muscle and a contracted one, in addition to allowing the muscles to rest. It is therefore important to relax the muscles between contractions, even if you do not feel the need to rest.

Frequency of Exercise Sessions

Exercising daily is recommended unless it is found to be too strenuous or fatiguing. In that case the exercises can be done every other day or at least three times a week. If you wish to undertake a long-term program to maintain optimum strength and endurance, continue to exercise with the optimum weight or a slightly reduced weight two to three times a week.

Equipment

A professional-type barbell set should be used. The set must include two safety locking collars, comfortable grip, preferably made of rubber, and a lightweight bar (solid steel bars are too heavy). The total weight of the bar, collars and handle should not exceed 1½ pounds.

The set should include the following weight plates: two plates each weighing ⅝, 1¼, and 2½ pounds (junior set), and two additional 2½- or 5-pound plates (adult set).

EXERCISE SELECTION GUIDE

Goal	Recommended Exercises	Optional Exercises
Strengthen all arm and shoulder muscles, prevent strains and injuries	Basic strengthening program, exercises 1 through 10	10A and 10B
Strengthen the grip and wrist	Exercises 1 and 2	
Strengthen the wrist and forearm	Exercises 3 and 4	

Goal	Recommended Exercises	Optional Exercises
Strengthen the elbow	Exercises 5 and 6	
Strengthen all shoulder and shoulder girdle muscles	Exercises 7, 8, 9 and 10	10A and 10B
Prevent/treat tennis elbow	Exercises 1, 2, 3, 4, 5, 6, 7, 8, 9, 10, 11, 12 and 12A	
Prevent/treat shoulder injuries	Exercises 7, 8, 9, 10, 13, 14, 15 and 16	10A and 10B 1, 2, 3, 4, 5 and 6

Basic Arm and Shoulder Exercises

STRENGTHENING EXERCISES

Exercise 1
Grip and Wrist Flexion

PURPOSE: To strengthen forearm and hand muscles that grip the racket and control wrist movement toward the palm of the hand.

EFFECT ON TENNIS: Developing a firm, yet relaxed grip. Improving control and strength of the wrist during all forehand strokes, service and overhead.

PROCEDURE: Place arm in starting position, palm up (photo 1a). Bend wrist up and hold for 6 seconds (photo 1b). Return to starting position. Rest 3–6 seconds. Repeat 10 times.

PROGRESSION: Use bar, handle and collars during the first session. Hold the bar the same way you hold a tennis racket, placing the thumb between the middle and index fingers. If able to complete ten repetitions with ease, increase the weight by 1¼ pounds during the following session. Do not increase weight at any level, if you feel undue pain or strain either during or after the exercise. Continue to gradually increase the weight until optimum level is reached (see photos below).

OPTIMUM WEIGHTS:

Men: 8–12 pounds.	Women: 4–8 pounds.
Boys: 4–10 pounds.	Girls: 3–6 pounds.

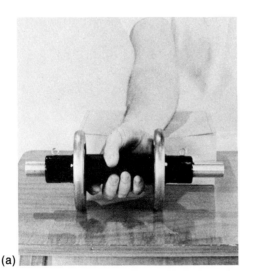

(a)

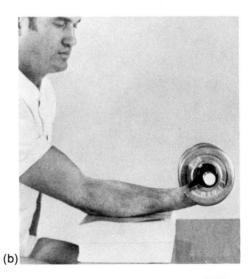

(b)

Exercise 2
Grip and Wrist Extension

PURPOSE: To strengthen the muscles that grip the racket and control wrist movement toward the back of the hand.

EFFECT ON TENNIS: Developing a firm, yet relaxed grip. Improving control and strength of wrist during all backhand strokes.

PROCEDURE: Place arm in starting position, palm down (photo 2a). Bend wrist up and hold for 6 seconds (photo 2b). Return to starting position. Rest 3–6 seconds. Repeat 10 times.

PROGRESSION: Same as for exercise 1.

OPTIMUM WEIGHTS: Men: 7–11 pounds. Women: 3–7 pounds.
 Boys: 3–9 pounds. Girls: 2–5 pounds.

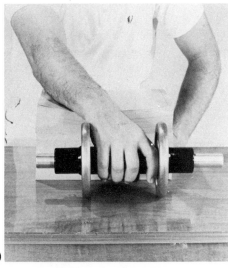

(a)

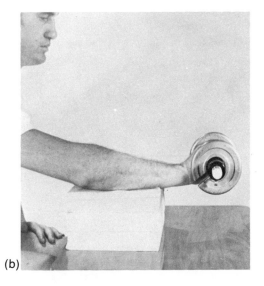

(b)

Exercise 3
Forearm Rotation—Supination

PURPOSE: To strength the muscles that rotate the forearm clockwise (right-handed persons), as well as the muscles responsible for gripping the racket during all backhand strokes, particularly the thumb muscles.

EFFECT ON TENNIS: Improved control and strength of the forearm and wrist during all backhand strokes. Firm backhand grip.

PROCEDURE: Place arm in starting position (photo 3a). (In case of pain, keep elbow at ninety degrees.) Rotate forearm clockwise, bringing bar to horizontal position, and hold for 6 seconds (photo 3b). Return to starting position. Rest 3–6 seconds. Repeat 10 times.

PROGRESSION: Use bar, handle, collars and a 1¼-pound weight during the first session. Use a backhand grip to hold the bar. If able to complete ten repetitions with ease, increase the weight by 1¼ pounds during the following session. Do not increase weight if you feel undue pain or strain either during or after the exercise. Continue gradually to increase the weight until optimum level is reached (see figures below).

OPTIMUM WEIGHTS (not including barbell assembly—bar, handle, collars):

Men: 5–10 pounds.	Women: 3–7 pounds.
Boys: 3–8 pounds.	Girls: 2–5 pounds.

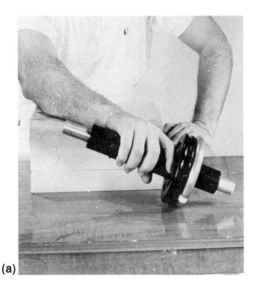

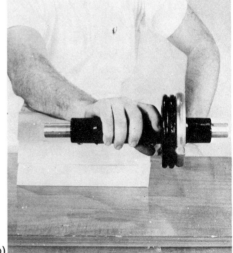

(a)　　　　　　　　　　　　　　　　(b)

Exercise 4
Forearm Rotation—Pronation

PURPOSE: To strengthen the muscles that rotate the forearm counterclockwise (right-handed persons), as well as the muscles responsible for gripping the racket during all the forehand strokes.

EFFECT ON TENNIS: Improved control and strength of the forearm and wrist during all forehand strokes. Firm forehand grip.

PROCEDURE: Place arm in starting position (photo 4a). (See exercise 3.) Rotate forearm counterclockwise, bringing bar to horizontal position, and hold for 6 seconds (photo 4b). Return to starting position. Rest 3–6 seconds. Repeat 10 times.

OPTIMUM WEIGHTS: Same as for exercise 3.

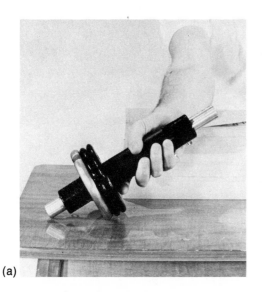

(a)

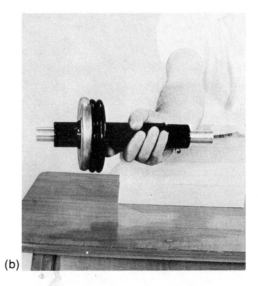

(b)

Exercise 5
Elbow Extension and Wrist Ulnar Deviation

PURPOSE: To strengthen the muscles that straighten the elbow as well as the muscles that bend the wrist toward the little finger.

EFFECT ON TENNIS: Controlled and firm elbow action during all backhand strokes. Strong, yet relaxed, elbow and wrist snap during service and overhead strokes. Quick and strong elbow extension during forehand and backhand volleys (punching the ball). Firm service and overhead grips.

PROCEDURE: Sit erect in chair, hold arm in starting position (photo 5a). Slowly extend elbow upward, pointing bar toward ceiling (photo 5b). Return to starting position. Rest 3–6 seconds. Repeat 10 times.

Alternate Method: (to be used if above method causes elbow pain). Lie along the edge of a bed and place your arm in starting position (photo 5c). Extend elbow (avoid full extension if painful), hold 3–6 seconds (photo 5d). Return to starting position. Rest 3–6 seconds. Repeat 10 times.

PROGRESSION: Use bar, handle and collars during first session. Use a service grip to hold the bar. If able to complete 10 repetitions with ease, increase weight by 1¼ pounds in the next session. Do not increase weight if you feel undue pain or strain either during or after the exercise. Continue to increase the weight gradually until optimum level is reached (see photos below).

OPTIMUM WEIGHTS: Men: 5–10 pounds.   Women: 3–7 pounds.
                      Boys: 3–8 pounds.   Girls: 2–5 pounds.

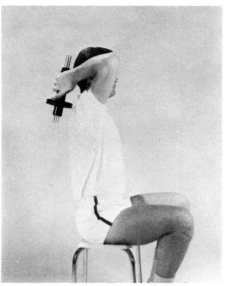

(a)

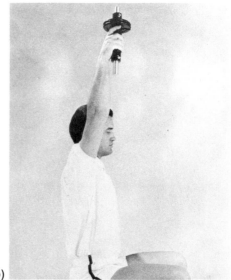

(b)

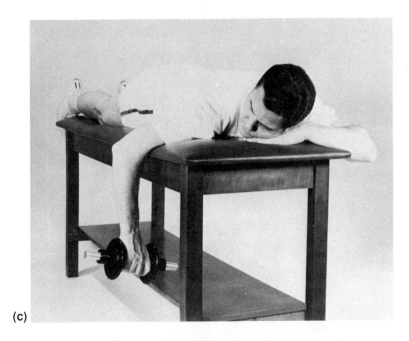

(c)

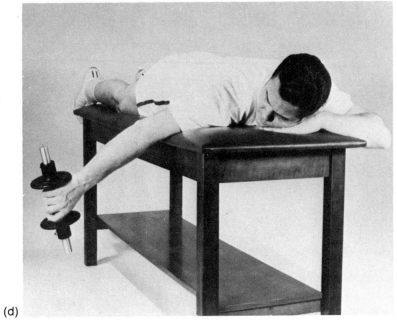

(d)

Exercise 6
Elbow Flexion

PURPOSE: To strengthen the muscles that bend the elbow.

EFFECT ON TENNIS: Improved elbow control.

PROCEDURE: Sit erect in chair and hold arm in starting position (photo 6a). Bend your elbow all the way up (photo 6b) and slowly return to starting position. Rest 3–6 seconds. Repeat 10 times.

PROGRESSION: Use bar, handle and collars during the first session. Increase by 1¼ pounds, if able to complete 10 repetitions with ease. Continue to increase the weight gradually until optimum level is reached (see photos below).

OPTIMUM WEIGHTS: Men: 10–15 pounds.   Women: 6–10 pounds.
                  Boys: 6–12 pounds.   Girls: 4–8 pounds.

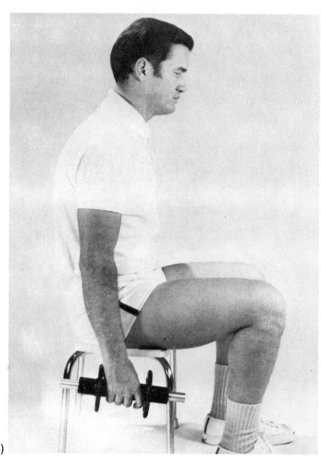

(a)

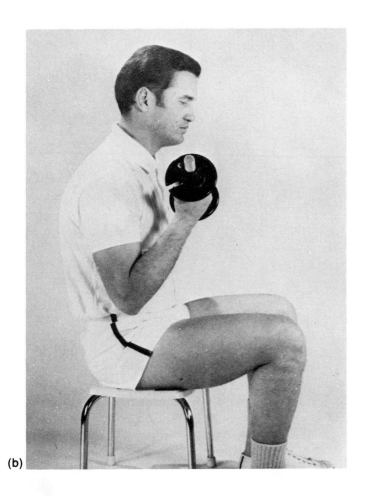

(b)

Exercise 7
Shoulder Flexion and Extension

PURPOSE: To strengthen the muscles that control forward (flexion) and back (extension) movements of the upper arm.

EFFECT ON TENNIS: Improved control and power of upper arm during low forehand and backhand strokes, and high backhand strokes.

PROCEDURE: Sit erect in chair, arm hanging down (photo 7a). Slowly raise arm forward (photo 7b), and all the way up (photo 7c). Slowly lower arm to starting position. Pull arm back as far as you can (photo 7d). Return to starting position. Rest 3–6 seconds. Repeat 10 times.

PROGRESSION: Use bar, handle and collars during the first session. If able to complete 10 repetitions with ease, increase the weight by 1¼ pounds during the following session. Do not increase weight if you feel undue strain or pain either during or after the exercise. Continue to gradually increase the weight until optimum level is reached (see photos below).

OPTIMUM WEIGHTS:	Men: 5–10 pounds.	Women: 3–7 pounds.
	Boys: 3–8 pounds.	Girls: 2–5 pounds.

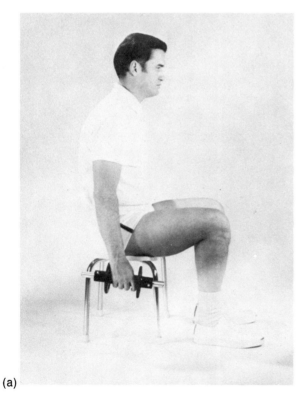

(a)

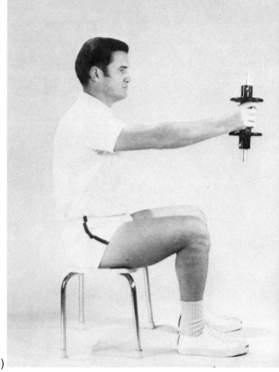

(b)

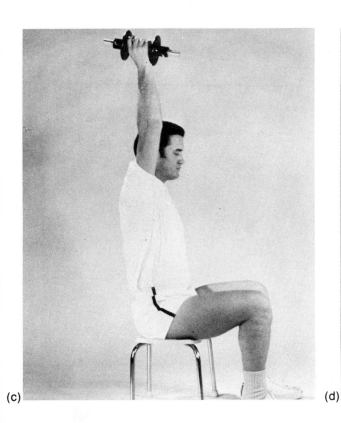

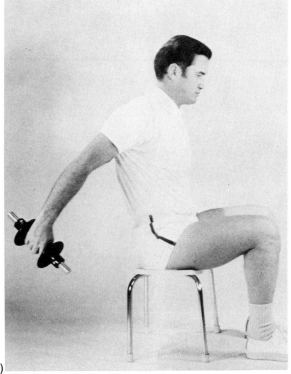

(c)

(d)

Exercise 8
Shoulder Abduction

PURPOSE: To strengthen the shoulder and shoulder girdle muscles that raise the upper arm sideways and up.

EFFECT ON TENNIS: Improved control and strength of the upper arm during backhand strokes as well as during high forehand, service and overhead.

PROCEDURE: Sit erect in chair, arm hanging down, palm of hand facing your body (photo 8a). Keeping your elbow straight, slowly raise your arm sideways to shoulder level, rotate palm up toward ceiling (photo 8b), then continue to raise the arm up until it touches the side of your head (photo 8c). Slowly lower arm sideways to shoulder level, rotate palm down and return to starting position. Rest 3–6 seconds. Repeat 10 times.

PROGRESSION AND OPTIMUM WEIGHTS: Same as for exercise 7.

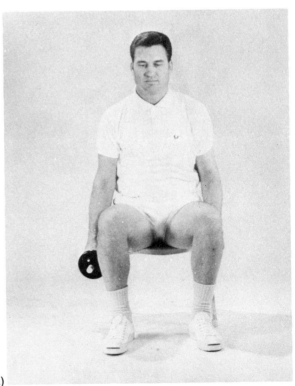

(a)

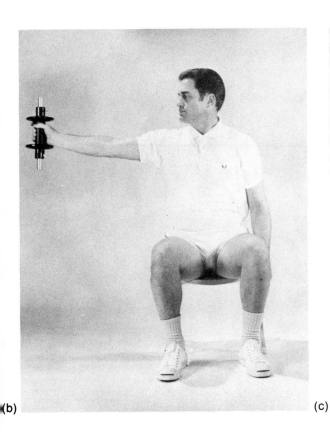

(b)

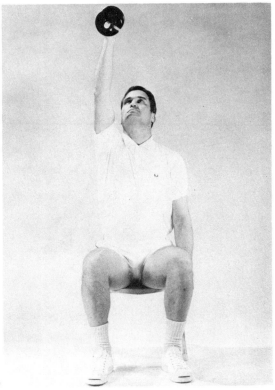

(c)

Exercise 9
Shoulder Internal and External Rotation

PURPOSE: To strengthen the muscles that rotate the upper arm in (internal rotation) and out (external rotation).

EFFECT ON TENNIS: Improved control and power of upper arm during all forehand strokes, service and overhead (internal rotation), as well as during all backhand strokes (external rotation).

PROCEDURE: Lie on your back, upper arm at shoulder level, elbow bent at ninety degrees (photo 9a). Roll your arm forward and down, until the forearm rests on the floor (photo 9b). Keep your elbow at shoulder level, do not permit it to slide down toward your hip. Slowly roll arm back all the way until the forearm touches the floor above the shoulder (photo 9c). Return to starting position. Rest 3–6 seconds. Repeat 10 times.

PROGRESSION AND OPTIMUM WEIGHTS: Same as for exercise 7.

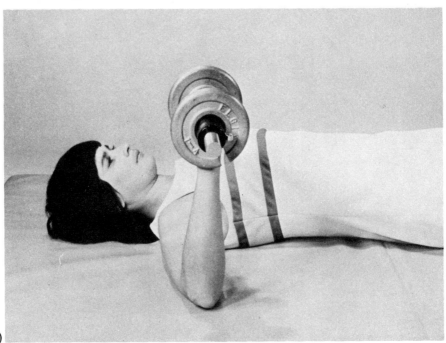

(a)

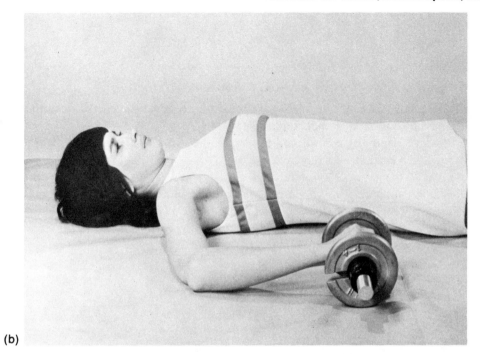

(b)

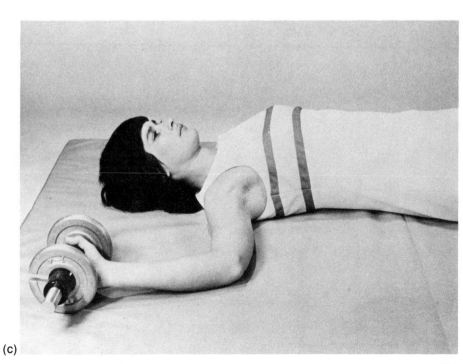

(c)

Exercise 10
Shoulder Horizontal Adduction and Abduction

PURPOSE: To strengthen the muscles that move the arm across the shoulders (horizontal adduction) and back (horizontal abduction).

EFFECT ON TENNIS: Improved control and power of the arm during forehand strokes (adduction) and backhand strokes (abduction).

PROCEDURE: Lie on your back, arm stretched sideways at shoulder level (photo 10a). Keeping your elbow straight, bring your arm across your shoulders (photo 10b), toward the opposite shoulder, permitting the elbow to bend slightly (photo 10c). Straighten your elbow and return slowly to starting position. Rest 3–6 seconds. Repeat 10 times.

PROGRESSION AND OPTIMUM WEIGHTS: Same as for exercise 7.

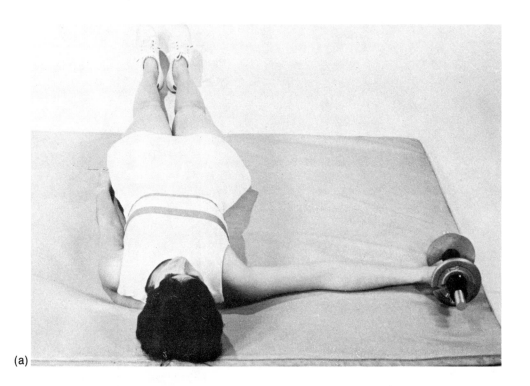

(a)

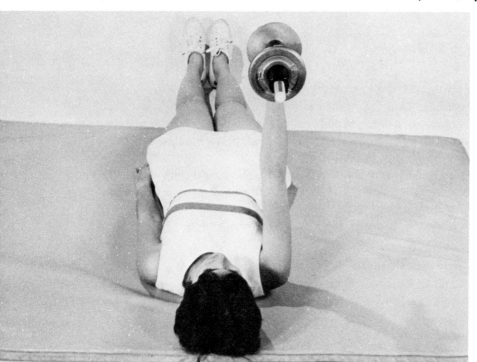

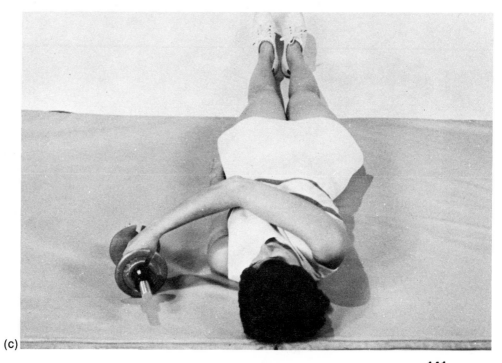

(c)

Exercise 10A
Optional

Similar to exercise 10, but arm is placed at a 45-degree angle above shoulder level (photo 10d), and from that position it is moved diagonally across the body and down until it reaches the floor on the other side of the body, at a 45-degree angle below shoulder level (photo 10e), and then returned to starting position.

EFFECT ON TENNIS: Improved control and power of the shoulder during service, overhead, high forehand, high forehand volley and underspin forehand, as well as low backhand, topspin backhand and topspin backhand lob.

PROGRESSION AND OPTIMUM WEIGHTS: Same as for exercise 7.

Note: At a later stage, you can try this exercise with the weights placed at one end of the bar (see exercises 3, 4 and 5). This will improve your wrist control.

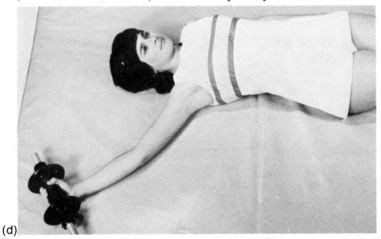

(d)

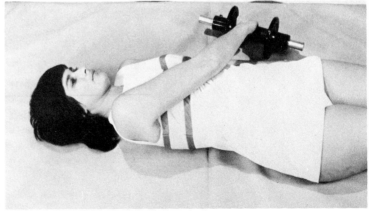

(e)

Exercise 10B
Optional

Similar to exercise 10A, but with the arm placed at a 45-degree angle below shoulder level (photo 10f), and from that position it is moved diagonally across the body and up, until it reaches the floor on the other side of the body at a 45-degree angle above shoulder level (photo 10g). The arm is then returned slowly to the starting position.

EFFECT ON TENNIS: Improved control and power of the shoulder during low forehand, topspin forehand and topspin forehand lob, as well as during high backhand volley and underspin backhand.

PROGRESSION AND OPTIMUM WEIGHTS: Same as for exercise 7.

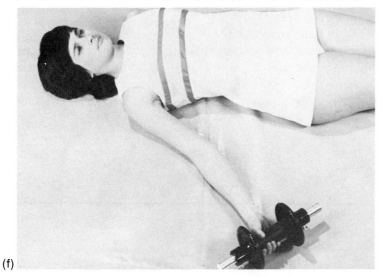

(f)

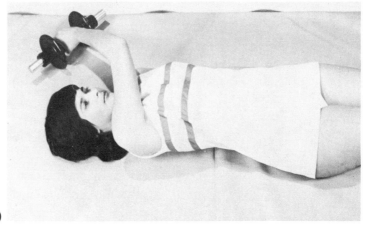

(g)

STRETCHING EXERCISES

Stretching exercises prevent muscle and tendon injuries and maintain joint flexibility. They are essential for relaxation, coordination and smoothness of movement.

In case of an injury, stretching should be done by a competent physical therapist and with the approval of a qualified physician.

Here are some stretching exercises that are particularly important to tennis players. Exercises 11, 12, and 12A will improve wrist and finger flexibility and help prevent injuries to the elbow, forearm and wrist. Exercises 13, 14, 15 and 16 will improve shoulder joint movements and prevent shoulder injuries.

Exercise 11
Wrist Extension

MUSCLES BEING STRETCHED: Wrist and finger flexors.

PROCEDURE: Place the palm of your hand flat on a table (photo 11a). Slowly move your arm toward your hand until you feel a mild stretch (photo 11b). Hold 3–5 seconds. Move your arm back and rest 3–5 seconds. Repeat 5–10 times.

NORMAL RANGE OF MOTION: 70 degrees or more (0 degrees—straight wrist).

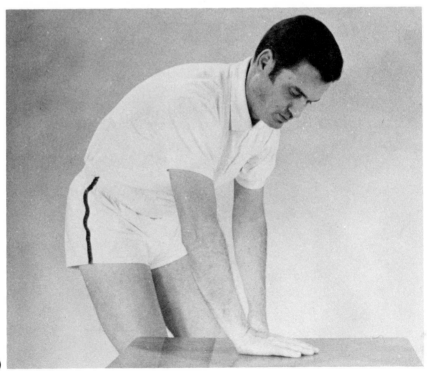

(a)

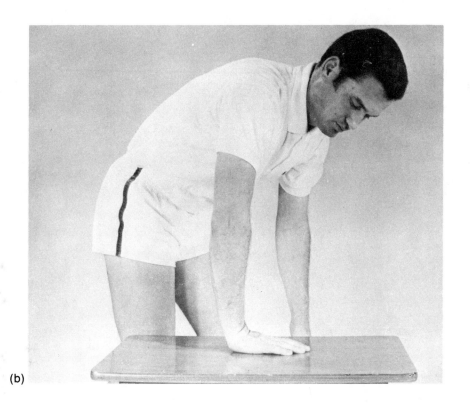

(b)

Exercise 12
Wrist Flexion

MUSCLES BEING STRETCHED: Wrist and finger extensors.

PROCEDURE:* Hold your right hand with left hand as shown (photo 12a). Slowly bend your right wrist until you feel a mild stretch (photo 12b). Do not overstretch. Hold 3–5 seconds. Release the pressure and rest 3–5 seconds. Repeat 5–10 times.

NORMAL RANGE OF MOTION: 70 degrees or more.

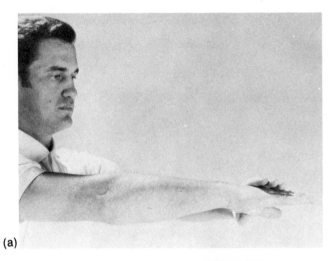

(a)

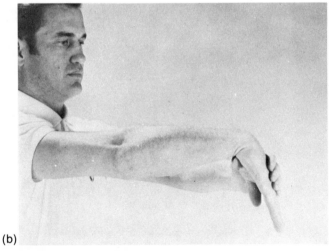

(b)

*Do both exercises first with elbow bent, later on with elbow straight.

Exercise 12A
Wrist Flexion with Ulnar Deviation

MUSCLES BEING STRETCHED: Wrist and finger extensors on the radial (thumb) side.
PROCEDURE:* Similar to exercise 12, but in addition, the wrist is bent toward the little finger until a mild stretch is felt (photo 12c).

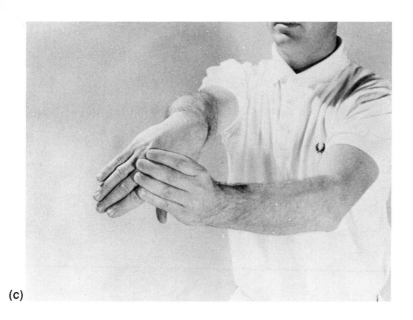

(c)

*Do both exercises first with elbow bent, later on with elbow straight.

Exercise 13
Shoulder Horizontal Adduction

MUSCLES BEING STRETCHED: Shoulder horizontal abductors.

PROCEDURE: Lying on your back, hold your right arm with your left hand above the elbow, and pull the right arm toward your chest until you feel a mild stretch (figure 13). Hold 3–5 seconds. Release pressure, and rest 3–5 seconds. Repeat 5–10 times.

NORMAL RANGE: Being able to bring upper arm under the chin.

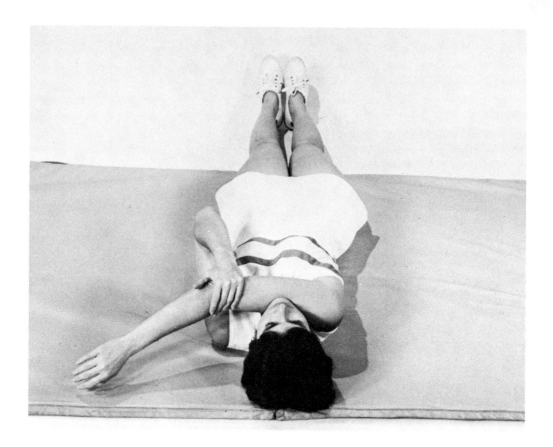

Exercise 14
Shoulder Internal Rotation

MUSCLES BEING STRETCHED: Shoulder external rotators.

PROCEDURE: Lying on your back, upper arm at shoulder level and elbow bent at ninety degrees, press your right forearm down with your left hand until you feel a mild stretch or forearm touches floor (figure 14). Hold 3–5 seconds. Release pressure, and rest 3–5 seconds. Repeat 5–10 times.

NORMAL RANGE: Being able to bring forearm down to floor with ease.

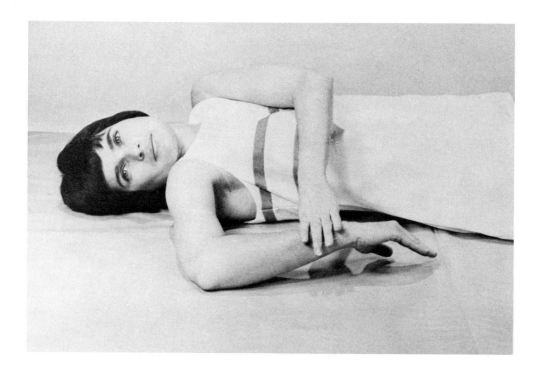

Exercise 15
Shoulder External Rotation

MUSCLES BEING STRETCHED: Shoulder internal rotators.
PROCEDURE: Similar to exercise 14, but in the opposite direction (figure 15).
NORMAL RANGE: Similar to exercise 14.

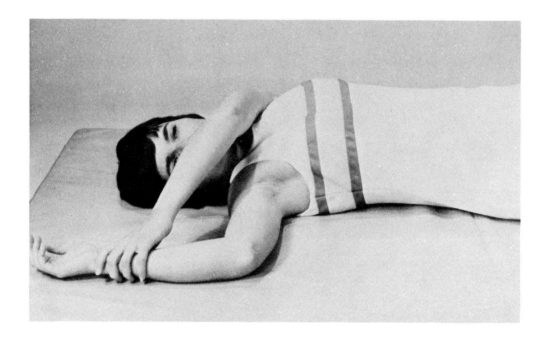

Exercise 16
Shoulder Flexion

MUSCLES BEING STRETCHED: Shoulder extensors.

PROCEDURE: Lying on your back and keeping your right elbow straight, push your right arm up over your head and down toward the floor (figure 16). Hold 3–5 seconds. Release pressure, and rest 3–5 seconds. Repeat 5–10 times.

NORMAL RANGE: Being able to bring arm down to floor with ease.

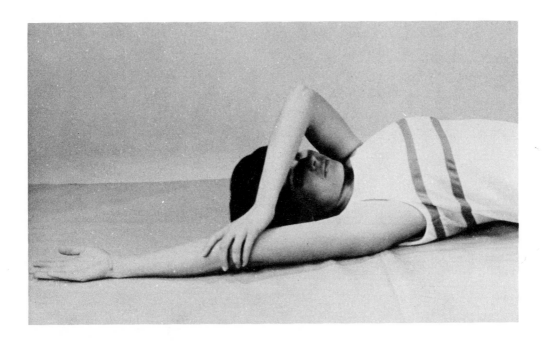

CHAPTER 8

Special Tips for Special Sports

Special Tips for Runners

In the chapter of this book dealing with "Prevention of Sports Injuries," runners are advised as to the selection of running shoes and running surfaces.

For many of us, running has become more than an avenue to cardio-respiratory fitness. It has become our sport. As a runner becomes more serious, he becomes more aware of the punishment to which he is forcing his feet and legs to adjust. As runners develop and begin road racing, this situation is aggravated. During a 26-mile marathon, a runner's feet each "pound the pavement" over sixteen thousand times. The stress of a road race, coupled with all the training it takes to get there, can cause serious leg and foot problems for the runner unless he employs an appropriate conditioning program as well as the right running shoe.

As usual, Dr. George Sheehan comes to the runner's rescue. He has developed a series of six exercises for runners which he calls "The Magic Six": three stretching exercises for the calf, hamstrings and the muscles of the lower back, and three strengthening exercises for the shin muscles, the thigh muscles and the abdomen. These exercises are being used by joggers and distance runners all over the country and they really do provide "trouble-free mileage," as Dr. Sheehan claims. Here are Dr. Sheehan's Magic Six:

1. Wall Pushup (to stretch calf muscle and Achilles tendon)

Starting position: Stand at arms' length from wall with palms against the wall.

Action:
(1) Lean in toward wall until a stretching sensation is felt in calf and Achilles tendon.
(2) Hold for 10 seconds.
(3) Return to starting position.

Suggested reps: Repeat above action for 1 minute.

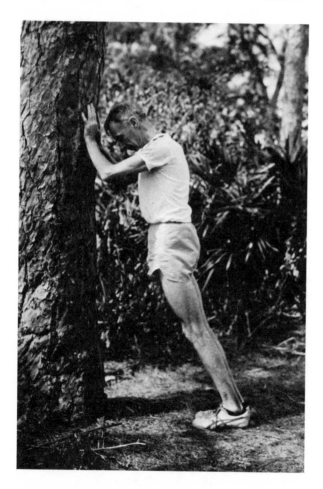

2. Hamstring Stretch

Starting position: Place right foot on a footstool or chair (begin with low elevation, raise as flexibility increases).

Action:
(1) Straighten leg and lock knee.
(2) With left leg kept straight, bring head toward knee of extended leg.
(3) Hold for 10 seconds.
(4) Straighten up to starting position.

Suggested reps: Repeat above action for 1 minute. Repeat complete sequence with leg positions reversed.

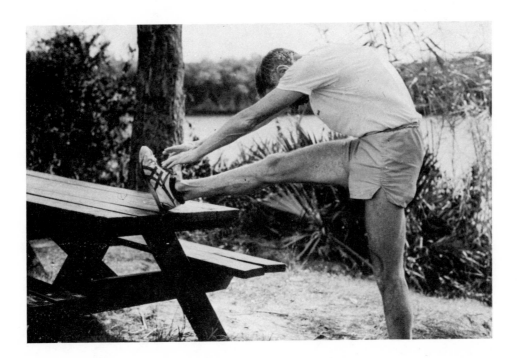

3. Backover for Hamstrings and Lower Back

Starting position: Lie on floor with legs extended.

Action:
(1) Bring straight legs over head.
(2) Try to touch floor with toes. Stretch toes toward floor until pain begins to be felt.
(3) Hold for 10 seconds.
(4) Relax by bending legs, bringing knees toward ears.

Suggested reps: Stretch and relax repeatedly for 1 minute.

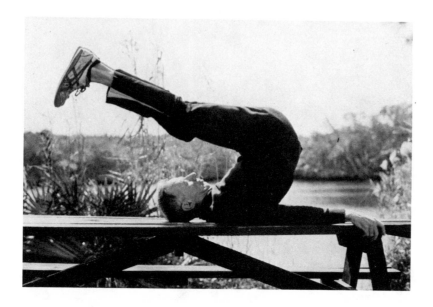

4. Shin Strengthener

Starting position: Sit on a table with legs hanging.

Action:
(1) Place 3–5-pound weight over toes of one foot. (You can place a dumbbell in a bucket.)
(2) Flex foot at ankle.
(3) Hold for 6 seconds.
(4) Relax.

Suggested reps: Flex and relax for 1 minute. Repeat sequence with other foot.

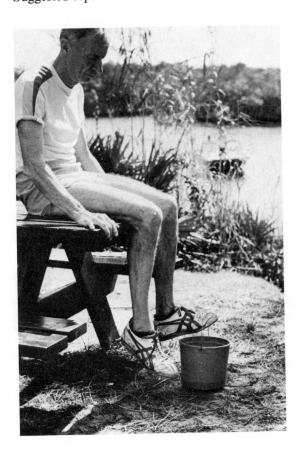

5. Thigh (quadriceps) Strengthener

Starting position: Same as for exercise 4 with weight.

Action:
(1) Flex leg at knee, causing leg to straighten.
(2) Hold for 6 seconds.
(3) Relax.

Suggested reps: Flex and relax for 1 minute. Repeat sequence using other leg.

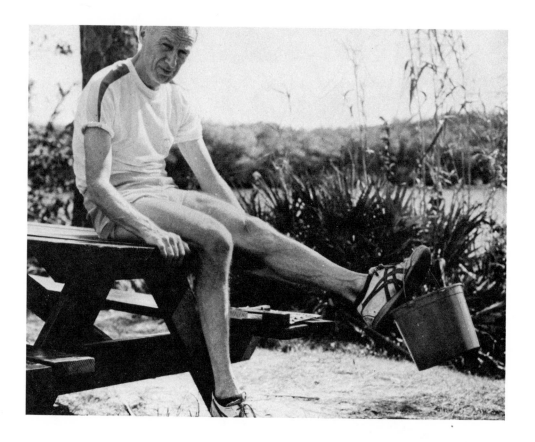

6. Bent-leg Sit-up

Starting position: Lie on floor with legs bent.

Action:
(1) Rise to a sitting position.
(2) Lie back.

Suggested reps: Dr. Sheehan advises trying to do at least 20, more if you can, fewer if you can't.

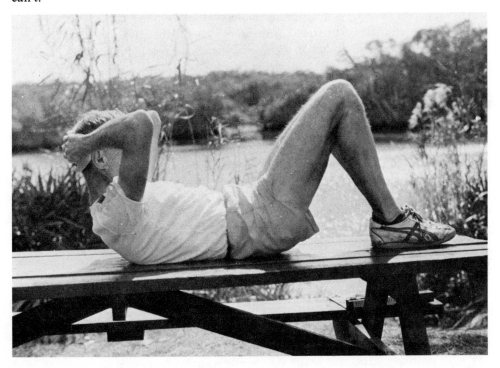

The Magic Six will only take you slightly more than six minutes. Try to do them before and after you run. This investment of twelve minutes of exercise will pay off with balanced muscular development in the legs, thighs, abdomen and lower back and, of prime importance to runners, a degree of protection from muscle pulls in these areas.

Special Tips for Skiers

Beginning downhill skiers do not find this sport to be very demanding in terms of cardio-respiratory endurance. Flexibility and leg strength are the more immediate concerns. As skill increases, skiing becomes more demanding physically and all aspects of fitness should be improved. It is especially important for the skier to keep his or her fitness program intact during the summer with added attention during the early fall, as the skiing season approaches.

Skiing is a sport that literally invites injury, but the risk of injury is dramatically reduced if the skier is conditioned. So don't show up on the ski trail without any physical preparation. If you make your training program a permanent year-round activity, you'll ski better and more confidently, have more fun on the slopes, reduce the risk of muscle pulls and strains, and you'll feel much better after a day of skiing.

FLEXIBILITY

Give special emphasis to flexibility in your workouts. This is the component of fitness that is going to give you the full range of body motion you'll want. It will contribute significantly to your agility and rhythm and it will help get you through a good many unexpected spills with damage restricted to the ego. Do as many as you can of the flexibility exercises illustrated in the chapter on "Warm-up and Flexibility Exercises." You'll notice that several of these routines, such as the hip rotators (exercise 9), have obvious association with the movements of skiing, but they're all important. Before buckling your skies on, do your regular warm-ups and try to add a few minutes of running in place or jogging.

ENDURANCE

It would be advisable for every skier to advance as far in the running program described in this book as he or she possibly can. First of all, it will make you a better athlete, and second, as your skiing skills improve and you get into some hard skiing, you'll want to have the physical stamina to handle it.

You've probably heard that many skiing injuries occur late in the day when skiers are tired. This seems to be true. It's one thing to know what you want your body to do—especially at high speed—but if your response is sluggish because of fatigue, you can easily get hurt. It's another reason to be fit.

As an adjunct to your regular running program, I'd like to recommend the following exercises.

This is one endurance-type exercise that is employed by just about all the World Class skiers. In addition to its endurance benefits, it also has flexibility and strength components. In the photos, Suzy Chaffee makes it look easy. It's not. You may want to try it using, at first, a very low foot stool but be sure you warm up first:

Bench Jump

Starting position: Stand alongside bench with feet together.

Action: Jump sideways over bench. Repeat, jumping from one side of the bench to the other.

Suggested reps and sets: This exercise will make sudden, severe demands on your cardio-respiratory system. Do as many reps as it takes to make you tired. Recover for 1 minute and repeat. You can gradually build up your tolerance for this exercise.

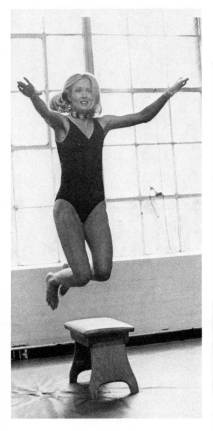
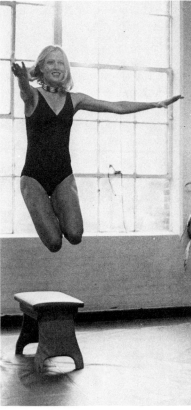
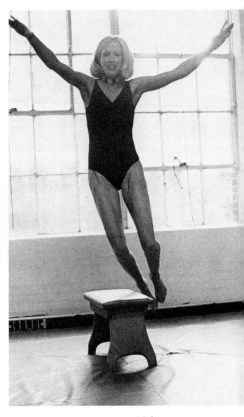

Rope Skipping

Here is another exercise from which skiers will benefit. It helps develop the type of muscular endurance that skiers require, as well as building cardio-respiratory endurance. A rope-skipping program is described in the "Endurance" chapter of this book.

Kangaroo Hop

This is one more exercise that can give skiers some desired spring in their legs.

Starting position: Stand erect with feet together.

Action: Leap upward, attempting to bring knees to chest.

Suggested reps: 2–3 sets of 10 reps, done as quickly as you can do them.

STRENGTH

Leg strength, of course, is of utmost importance to skiers. Make sure to do the leg exercises found in the "Strength Development" chapter. The *toe raises* and *half squats* will be especially helpful.

Upper body strength is also important in skiing. For good pole work, you'll need strong arms and shoulders. So don't neglect the pushups and other arm exercises in the "Strength" chapter.

Special Tips for Water Sports

In addition to competitive swimming, there are two water sports that call for a high degree of conditioning: surfing and scuba diving. Competitive swimming presupposes an adequate formal coaching program. I have included a complete program for competitive swimmers elsewhere in this book. This section will concern itself with those who are considering surfing and scuba diving as recreational activities.

SKIN DIVING AND SCUBA DIVING

If you are interested in skin diving or scuba (using Self Contained Underwater Breathing Apparatus) diving, physical fitness is not only desirable, it's a must. Exploring with a mask

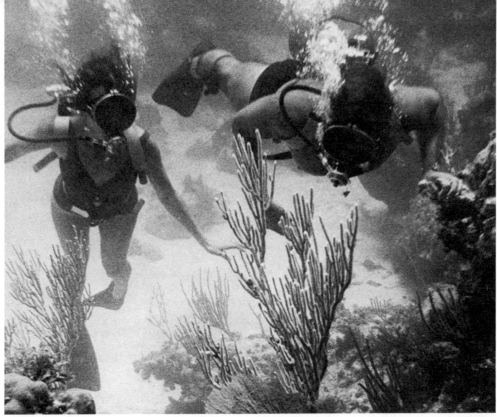

and a "snorkle" in four or five feet of water is one thing; but if you are going to get seriously involved in this sport, your fitness will be your money in the bank. In addition to your regular fitness workouts, the experts at the U.S. Army diving school at Fort Eustis, Virginia, recommend the following conditioning routines:

First, a beginner should be able to swim 220 yards on the surface of the water, using his own free style; 25 yards underwater, with two breaks of the water for air; swim 150 feet wearing ten pounds of weights; and tread water for 15 minutes.

Conditioning Programs for Cardio-respiratory Fitness.
1. Run 1 mile (absolute minimum) daily.
2. Swim continuously. Begin with 15 minutes and slowly work up to 1 to 1½ hours, 4 times a week.

Strength Program.
1. Pushups, 25 each workout—4 times a week.
2. Situps (bent leg), 50 each workout—4 times a week.
3. Half squats with barbell, 2 sets of 10. Begin with ½ body weight and work up—4 times a week.
4. Heel raises with barbell, 3 sets of 10. Begin with ½ body weight and work up—4 times a week.
5. Pullups, begin with 2 sets of 5 and work up to 5 sets of 8—4 times a week.

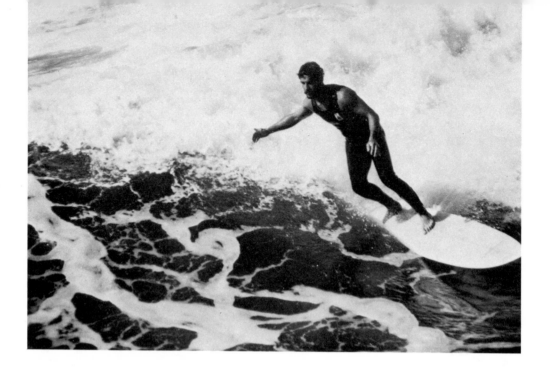

SURFING

All of the strength and endurance exercises suggested for scuba divers are highly recommended for surfers. You should be able to swim 100 yards all out and about 400 yards at a steady pace. And make sure you can meet these minimums in choppy water, because you won't be surfing in a swimming pool.

The leg exercises that appear above can be especially valuable for the surfer because he or she must be able to squat down and rise up quickly and easily on the board.

Here's an exercise for getting up on the surfboard. It was developed by William D. Nelson, a surfing instructor and author, and appears in his book *Surfing—A Handbook,* published by Aurback Publishing Company, Philadelphia, Pa. Do this exercise while lying on an imaginary surfboard on your living room rug:

1. Lie on the floor, face down as if you are paddling.
2. Put hands beside your chest.
3. With knees on the floor, lift the lower part of your legs and your feet to the perpendicular.
4. Push up with your arms, throw your back out and down, while jackknifing your torso and thighs.
5. Your body and legs should now be in mid-air, while you are momentarily balanced on your hands.
6. Bring your feet and legs up under you, so that your feet land one behind the other, each on the center line of your imaginary board.
7. Remove your hands from the floor and straighten up.
8. Having started out facing forward, you should now be facing 90 degrees away, or sideways, standing in a surfing position

This is an important exercise. You have to be able to get up on your surfboard without using your feet, which will be hanging off the end of the board. Do 10 repetitions of this routine as rapidly as you can. Do three sets with 30 seconds' rest between each set.

Special Tips for Hikers and Backpackers

I've included tips for hikers in this section because it's such a beguiling activity. In the springtime especially, thousands of people are lured out into the wilderness and the hiking trails. Sad to say, many of these people are not fit. They've got a good idea; but they're not prepared physically to follow it through. You don't get your legs, back and cardio-respiratory system ready for a strenuous hike when you are on the side of a mountain. It's too late then. And if you have your family with you, you've compounded the risk by a factor governed by the number of unfit people in your party. Your weekend of hiking and climbing in rough country is supposed to be fun. Don't make it into a catastrophe or, worse yet, a tragedy by neglecting the most essential piece of equipment: your personal fitness.

If you plan on tackling the hiking trails, you'd better begin right now on a full-scale conditioning program. There are going to be many physical activities that you are going to have to be able to do—most of them unexpected—and they are going to require strength, agility, fast reaction time and a good range of body motion, as well as cardio-respiratory endurance.

Most experienced hikers, climbers and backpackers I've spoken to agree that the flexibility, endurance and strength-development programs in this book are adequate for most hiking situations. Here are a few additional suggestions:

Endurance:
Add running stairs or steep hills to endurance activities.

Strength:
1. Give special attention to situps. If you're going to be carrying a pack on steep slopes try to work up to 50 reps, 4 times a week.
2. Work on heel raises with dumbbell. Try beginning with ½ body weight—3 sets of ten, 4 times a week.
3. Half squats with dumbbell, ½ body weight—3 sets of ten, 4 times a week.

If these weights are too heavy, use the amount of weight you can handle easily while accomplishing the recommended number of reps and sets.

CHAPTER 9

Advanced Programs for Competitive Athletes

While this book has been compiled mainly with the weekend athlete in mind, I am aware that many families with a Saturday tennis player or two also include at least one competitive athlete.

The scholastic football, basketball or baseball player is not a weekend sportsman and his physical capabilities and requirements are a lot different from Dad's. He is—or should be—just about peaking out physically. Should be! Many high school and college athletes never realize their potential because they never reach the level of fitness that could get them there.

The professional athletes we've spoken to realize this and, when they have opportunities to counsel boys and girls with goals in athletics, they stress the importance of fitness. Pat Fischer, the Washington Redskins' indestructible defensive back, assures young athletes that he's determined never to be beaten by an opponent because of being in inferior physical condition. And with sixteen years in the National Football League, it appears that his philosophy works for him. Defensive end Jim Marshall, of the Vikings, tells about his approach to conditioning: "I do as many as I can of each drill; then I do ten more. This assures me that, no matter how tired I am, I've always got something left." Redskins' quarterback Joe Theisman tells about being the last one to leave the practice field. He was recently quoted in the newspapers as saying, "If I'm competing for a position and my competitor works out for five hours, I'll work out for six."

Relief pitcher Tug McGraw, of the Philadelphia Phillies, believes that his running program gives him the stamina to do the job right up to the end of the season. "I can't claim to

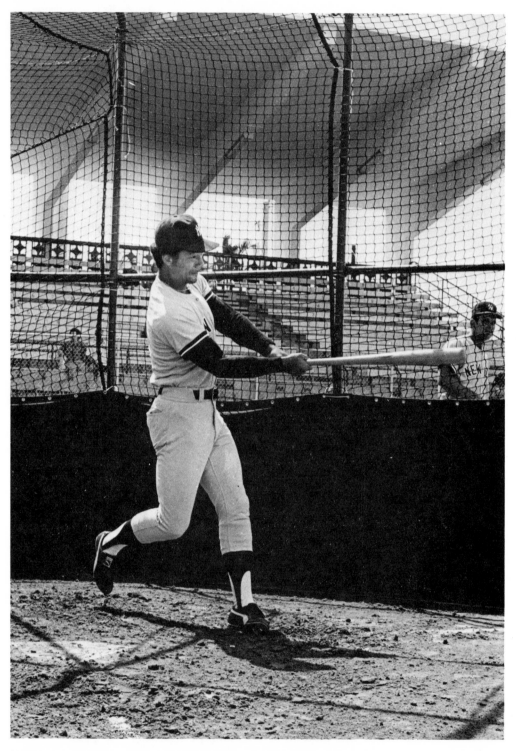

Yankee outfielder Roy White has a special program for strengthening arms, wrists and hands.

be one of those athletes who enjoys running," admits Tug, "but it's the most important part of my conditioning program. And sometimes, in a tough game situation, when I'm tired and I have to reach back for that special pitch, that's when it pays off."

Miler Marty Liquori, one of the great names in American track, has a formula: "I work so hard on my training and conditioning that—everything else being equal—I end up feeling I deserve to win."

Each of these athletes has established a subtle thread connecting physical and mental preparation. Get them talking about conditioning, and before you know it, they're talking about confidence. Many young athletes lack confidence. A fitness program can provide a base for confidence, because if you know that your body isn't going to let you down, you can concentrate on skill development.

The following programs were devised for young athletes by athletes who have achieved superstar status. Any athlete—even the weekend variety—can benefit by reading this section. It will reaffirm everything you've learned so far: especially that you get in shape to play—you don't play to get in shape.

Baseball

Roy White, the New York Yankees' veteran outfielder, has provided a useful, off-season program for scholastic baseball players. Softball players should take note of Roy's exercises for hands, wrists and forearms.

BASEBALL CONDITIONING
by Roy White, New York Yankees

STRONG HANDS, WRISTS AND FOREARMS

There are many ways to build strong hands, wrists and forearms. You can start by constantly squeezing a hard rubber ball, first with your throwing hand and then with your catching hand. Wrist curls with dumbbells will build strong forearms and wrists; be sure to do both forward and reverse curls, so that you avoid overdeveloping one set of arm muscles. You can stretch the arm muscles by hanging for 5 to 10 seconds from a horizontal bar (or a door, if you're working out in your home) and then loosen the arms up by playing catch. Do 3 sets of 10 to 15 repetitions with a 25-pound dumbbell at least 3 times a week to get the maximum benefit from arm curls.

Another exercise involves rolling a weight onto a broomstick. Fasten a 15-pound weight to the end of a rope and tie the other end of the rope to the center of a 15-inch broomstick. Extend your arms to the front parallel to the ground and slowly roll the weight up and down, winding the rope around the broomstick as you rotate your wrists. I begin this exercise in December with 3 sets of 5 repetitions and work up to 3 sets of 25 repetitions just prior to pre-season training (the start of spring training in mid-February). You should time this program to begin 10 weeks prior to the start of your baseball team's official practices and do the same repetitions as I do every day.

SWINGING A HEAVY BAT

Swinging a heavy bat can also build strong wrists, hands and forearms. The mild overload can greatly increase your bat speed, which is the key to better batting. Work with a bat that is 7 to 15 ounces heavier than your regulation bat. Do not use an extremely heavy bat (more than 15 ounces) because this causes the body's muscles to compensate for the heavy bat and you end up practicing an unnatural swinging motion. Concentrate on building the strength of the bottom hand on the bat; this is the hand that controls the speed of the bat during the swing. With a stronger, swifter bottom hand on the bat, you won't get jammed as often on inside fastballs and you will be able to wait longer before committing yourself to swing. Start with 25 swings in the early off-season and work up to 100 swings per day by the start of pre-season training. I begin in early December and reach the 100-swing plateau by the time I leave for spring training in mid-February. You should begin this exercise 10 weeks prior to the beginning of your official practices. A word of caution: don't swing too hard too soon; you will only slow your progress by causing blisters on your hands.

QUICKNESS AND SPEED

Superior quickness is a product of both mental and physical reactions. Physically, it is being able to move a short distance with grace, agility, speed and balance, such as an infielder's shuffle into position to field a ground ball. Brooks Robinson is a player with superior quickness on the field; next time you see him play, watch how fast he maneuvers into position. Mentally, he anticipates the flight of the ball from the moment it meets the bat; he concentrates on the swing of the batter and reacts to the crack of the bat instantaneously. Your feet should be in motion long before you judge the angle and speed of the ball.

Speed can be increased by maintaining good running form with the weight forward. You can improve your speed by practicing 30-yard sprints. Crouch in your leadoff position, cross over with your left foot to start and run as hard as you can for 30 yards. To maintain your speed in the off-season, play basketball. A good, hard game of basketball is filled with short bursts of speed, which will keep your legs in shape for the same type of movements in baseball. Off-season activity is important for keeping off extra weight, which will slow down your running speed. Report to spring practice in shape so that you can use the early and pre-season training time for sharpening baseball skills. Your year-round program should include situps, toe touches, hamstring stretches, leg lifts, pushups and running; in the off-season, you should work out no fewer than 3 times a week.

OFF-SEASON EXERCISE PROGRAM

Activity   *Frequency*

1. Running ....4 times per week, 15 minutes per day
2. Bent-knee situps ....4 times per week, 4 sets of 10 per day
3. Toe raises ....4 times per week, 3 sets of 10 per day
4. Side twisters ....4 times per week, 5 sets of 10 per day
5. Toe touches.........................4 times per week, 2 sets of 25 per day
6. Windmills............................4 times per week, 2 sets of 25 per day
7. Pushups (fingertip)...............4 times per week, 2 sets of 10 per day

Basketball

Basketball players competing on high school and college teams will find some valuable ideas in Gail Goodrich's training program. Gail has been one of the premier guards in the NBA for several years. His interest in physical fitness goes back to his UCLA years. He has developed his training program so that he can feel as strong and as ready to play on the last day of the season as on opening day.

Note: The training concepts used by basketball players have proven to be useful to volleyball players as well.

AGILITY AND ENDURANCE
by Gail Goodrich

REACTION DRILLS

To play guard, I knew I would have to have quick hands and coordinated movement of the feet. Here are the drills that I adopted to build quick reactions and coordination; they are the same drills that I teach athletes in basketball camps throughout the country. Try them and watch yourself improve too.

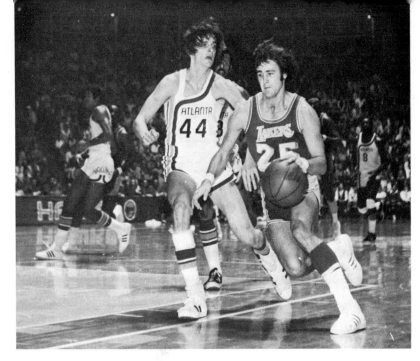

Gail Goodrich as a Los Angeles Laker. (UPI)

For building quick hands:

- Place your hands behind your back, lean over and have your teammate hold the basketball at eye level, two feet in front of you. Have him drop the ball without warning and try to catch it before it hits the floor.
- Hold the basketball between your legs, slightly spread in the crouched position, the right hand grasping the ball from behind and the left hand from the front. Let go of the ball, reverse your hands, and catch the ball before it hits the floor.

For building quick feet:

- Assume the customary defensive position, your feet spread slightly more than shoulder-width apart in the crouched stance. Have your teammate hold the basketball chest-high and move it either left or right. React to his shifting of the ball by shuffling quickly in the direction that he chooses. Don't cross your feet, but move them together, then apart, as you shuffle laterally. Continue the drill for one minute. Rest 30 seconds and repeat 4 more times.

For building coordination:

- Take two basketballs and tap them simultaneously against the backboard. Set a goal of 25 consecutive taps and increase by 10 each day.

IMPORTANCE OF ENDURANCE

You cannot improve your skills in basketball unless you've achieved a sound fitness base with strong legs. Running is the best way to achieve this base. I like to run barefoot on grassy terrain because the slight "give" of the turf forces the ankle joint to constantly flex and adjust, thus strengthening the ligaments—which helps guard against sprains during regular season play.

Here's my pre-season running program, which I have been following since it was first designed for me at UCLA. I recommend that you begin the program eight weeks prior to the first day of official practice. At UCLA I would run a 508-yard hill every other day; this made the program a little tougher and it was a change of pace from running over flat, grassy terrain. Either way you slice it, this program is a good conditioner and it will get you ready for the season. I average 40 minutes a game. To prepare for this, I work up to 30 consecutive minutes of daily running during my 8-week pre-season training program.

GAIL GOODRICH'S PRE-SEASON RUNNING PROGRAM

Week No.	Length of Time Running
1	10 minutes
2	12 minutes
3	15 minutes
4	18 minutes
5	21 minutes
6	24 minutes
7	27 minutes
8	30 minutes

You should run at least 5 times per week to gain maximum benefit from the gradual increase of time spent running.

SUPPLEMENTARY DRILLS TO BUILD LEG STRENGTH

To increase leg strength for jumping, try running and hopping the bleachers that flank your football field. Here's a good workout to supplement your 8-week running program:

Bleacher drill (same drill can be done with staircase in high rise building):

- Run 50 rows, hop 10, walk down. Repeat 5 times, 3 times per week.
- Increase 10 rows running and 5 rows hopping each week until you're running 120 rows and hopping 45 rows for each repetition (8th week).

Rim-touch drill:

- From standing start, jump and touch the rim 10 consecutive times with your right hand. Then repeat with your left hand.
- From a running start, jump and touch the rim 10 consecutive times with both hands.

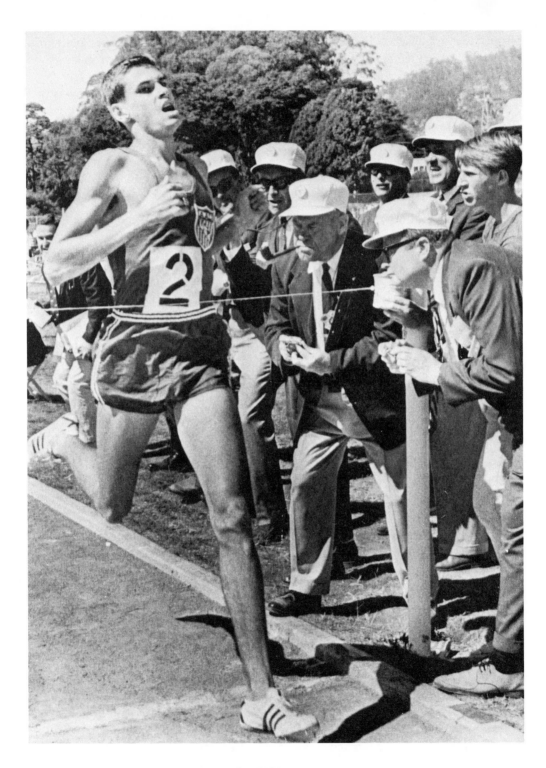

Jim Ryun sets World record for the mile. (UPI)

DISTANCE RUNNING
by Jim Ryun

If you think the mile run is your challenge, you are going to have to put yourself on a long-range training program. I have developed a year-round routine that is specially geared to scholastic athletes. It is designed to get the miler started slowly during the summer break and bring him to a peak of readiness for the spring competitive season.

July: Long, easy runs one hour a day. No particular pace. (This is a good time for high-school milers to begin building a good endurance base for the cross country season that begins in September.)

August: Same as July.

September: Two workouts a day. Five to 7 miles in the morning at a leisurely pace. Ten to 15 miles in the afternoon.

October: Same as September, but add Fartlek (Swedish term meaning speed/play). Fartlek is a natural and enjoyable training routine that is done away from the track and calls for continuous running at various speeds, if possible over a soft, springy surface.

November and December: Same routines as September and October, with periodic interval training that mixes routines such as 10 repeat miles with 2½-minute resting periods, or 2 or 3 repeat two-miles with 2½-minute resting periods with afternoon runs. Also, this is when I vary my workouts by running on the track to drive the monotony out of the running. For example, I'll go to the track and run several ½ miles or ¾ miles or ¼ miles twice a week. On one day during the week, usually Sunday, I'll run only once and it will be a continuous workout for maybe 20 miles. Average miles per week is 100 to 120.

January, February and March: Still averaging 100 miles per week, but the emphasis in the workouts is now on speed. Repeat 100's, 220's, 440's, 660's and 880's are performed at race tempo or better.

April, May and June: Workouts are to gain sharpness. Race tempo runs are done on Monday and Tuesday of week when meet is on Saturday. A typical workout during the competitive outdoor season is (1) warmup, (2) run a ¾ mile, (3) jog a ½ mile, (4) run a ½ mile, (5) jog a ½ mile, (6) run a 660, (7) jog ½ mile and then (8) run a ¼ mile. The emphasis is entirely on speed. Taper off the running drills on Wednesday and Thursday and jog on Friday, the day before the meet.

WEIGHT-LIFTING EXERCISES

Athletes vary as to the amount of weight that they can reasonably handle; two boys the same age and size do not necessarily have the same capacity and ability to lift weights. For this reason I hesitate to prescribe a set of exercises with specific repetitions that every high-school miler should follow. The definitive weight program just doesn't exist. Each athlete must find his relative starting point and work up from there. Below are listed some of the exercises that have helped me along the way. If you wish to apply them to your training program, consult with your coach concerning how they are done, frequency of workouts, number of repetitions and the weight resistance to be used.

- Forward arm curls.
- Reverse arm curls.
- Military press.
- Bench press.
- Half squats.
- Toe raises.
- Tricep curls.
- Upright curls.
- Upright lifts.
- Hamstring extensors.
- Knee lifts.

Football

For most sports fans, the name Roger Staubach epitomizes the word "competitor." Young men engaged in high-school or college football, could have few better examples on which to pattern their development as athletes than the fine quarterback of the Dallas Cowboys. Certainly, few athletes have been able to catalog and articulate the components of their success as well as Roger. Near the top of his list is physical conditioning.

MY 8-WEEK PRE-SEASON TRAINING PROGRAM
by Roger Staubach

I prepare myself physically year-round to compete; also I develop myself mentally to win. It is extremely important that you believe inside that you've worked as hard as possible. Then, mentally, you know you can do your job.

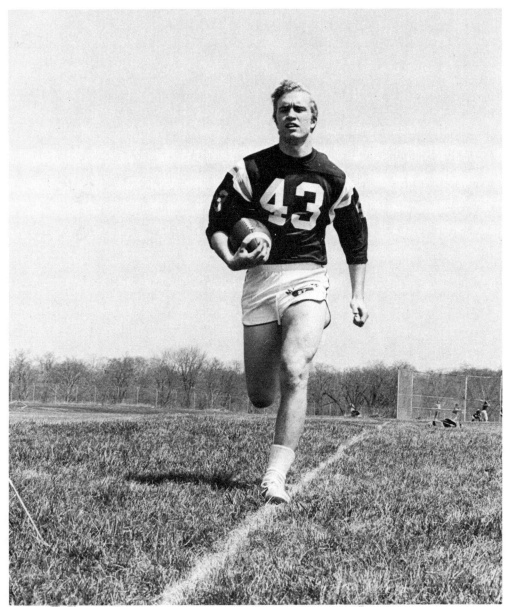

Roger Staubach's program is designed for high school and college athletes.

Each individual on a team has got to strive for his physical peak. Then he will be emotionally ready, too. You've got to be ready to give that extra five minutes, when practice is over, running those hundred-yard sprints. If one or two men in key positions slack off, it can be the difference between a win or loss in the game. Careful physical and mental preparation is what makes a successful team. Try this 8-week conditioning program prior to the beginning of fall football practice.

8-WEEK PRE-SEASON TRAINING PROGRAM

| | | | Total Mileage | | | |
| | | | Endurance | | Speed | |
Week No.	Daily Activity	Target Time	Daily	Weekly	Daily	Weekly*
1	Jog and run 1½ miles.	10–12 min.	1½	7½	0	0
2	Jog and run 2 miles.	13–15 min.	2	10	0	0
3	Jog and run 3 miles.	18–23 min.	3	15	0	0
4	Run 2 miles and recover by walking ¼–½ mile.	10–12 min.	2	10	0	0
	Jog 1 mile.	7–9 min.	1	5	0	0
5	Run 1½ mile and recover by walking ¼–½ mile.	8–10 min.	1½	7½	0	0
	Run 880 yards, 3 reps. Recover by jogging ½ mile.	2½–3 min.	0	0	1	5
6	Run 1 mile and recover by walking ¼–½ mile.	5–7 min.	1	5	0	0
	Run 880 yards, 3 reps.	2¼–2½ min.	0	0	1½	7½
7	Jog 1 mile.	7–9 min.	1	5	0	0
	Run 880 yards, 2 reps. Recover by walking ¼–½ mile between each rep.	2–2½ min.	0	0	1	5
	Run 440 yards, 4 reps. Recover by walking ¼–½ mile between each rep.	65–75 sec.	0	0	1	5
	Run 220 yards, 2 reps. Recover by walking ¼–½ mile between each rep.	2–2½ min.	0	0	½	2½
8	Jog 1 mile.	7–9 min.	1	5	0	0
	Run 220 yards, 2 reps. Recover by walking 100 yards between each rep.	25–28 sec.	0	0	¼	1¼
	Run 440 yards, 2 reps. Recover by walking ¼ mile between each rep.	50–58 sec.	0	0	½	2½
	Run 100 yards, 4 reps. Recover by walking 200 yards between each rep.	9.8–10.8 sec.	0	0	¼	1¼
	Run 40 yards, 10 reps.	5.0–5.8 sec.	0	0	¼	1¼

*Based upon 5 workouts per week.

Soccer

THE WAY TO GOOD SOCCER: RUN, RUN, RUN!
by Gordon Bradley, Coach of
the New York Cosmos Soccer Team

If you want to play soccer, you must be prepared to run—but not without the soccer ball. You cannot play this game unless you are able to run for long periods of time, sometimes in game conditions as long as 20 minutes without a rest at nearly full speed. In addition, if you cannot control the soccer ball with your feet, your running ability and endurance are wasted. Running, of course, builds strong legs, which not only power you up and down field, but also provide the necessary means for kicking the ball.

THE SHUTTLE RUN

The key to building both endurance for running the full length of a game and skillful ball control is to practice the shuttle run, a drill that combines both cardio-vascular training and dribbling with all-out bursts up and down the soccer field. This drill is best performed in 3-man teams drawn from the full soccer squad; divide into 3-man teams with each team having a good mix of fast and slow men, in order to make the competition even. Set out 6 flags at 15-yard intervals, placing the first flag at the 15-yard line at one end of the soccer field and the last one at the 90-yard line at the other end of the field.

The object of the drill is for each team to try and run the course 6 times in the fastest possible time. Each player will have to dribble the ball as fast as possible up to the flags, around them and back to the starting point.

In repetition 1, the first player must dribble the ball around the 15- and 60-yard markers; in repetition 2, he must dribble the ball around the 30- and 75-yard markers; and in repetition 3, he must dribble the ball around the 45- and 90-yard markers. Repetitions 4 through 6 repeat the first 3 repetitions. This drill should be done without stopping and at the fastest possible speed. In just a very short time, you will pick up speed in dribbling and improve ball control with the feet.

CIRCUIT TRAINING

Overall fitness is a tremendous asset to a soccer player. For this reason, I recommend circuit training; that is, a series of exercises and routines that alternately stress different

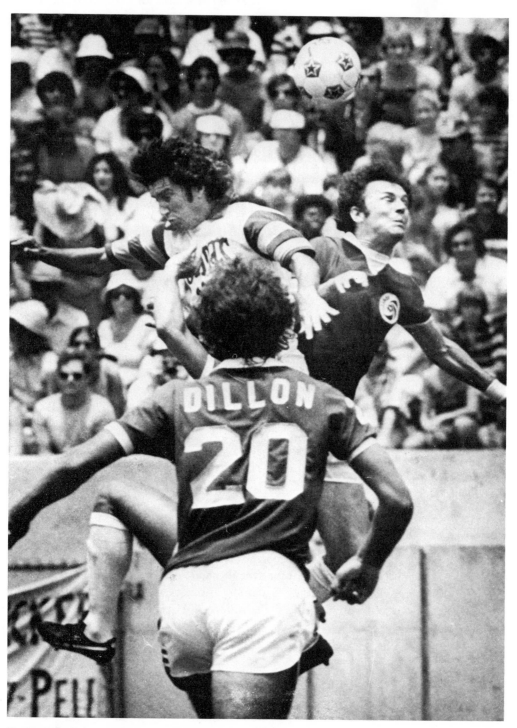

Franz Beckenbauer gets off a head shot during his first game as a member of the New York Cosmos. (UPI)

systems and muscles of the body. For example, a player might do 20 pushups and then run 10-yard sprints up and down the soccer field. The pushups work on the muscular-skeletal development of the shoulders and arms, while the sprints increase the efficiency of the cardio-vascular system. This is the essence of a properly designed circuit: one system working while another rests. I employ a variety of drills and exercises, such as rope climbing, sprinting, situps, stepping up and down from a bench. Pick your own mix of exercises, but be sure to alternate the muscles and systems that are being taxed on each successive exercise. Design a circuit of exercises that takes 15 minutes to complete at first try; then work to complete these same exercises in 12 minutes or better.

OFF-SEASON TRAINING

It is easy to practice on your own. All you need is a ball and a wall and you can practice kicking, heading and shooting. Practice dribbling and changing direction. Learn to kick with either foot. Work out with a friend and take turns trying to dribble the ball around each other. This is an excellent drill because it simulates the pressure that you will receive in a game.

And if there is a substitute for practice, it's playing. So, join a sand-lot team in the off-season and play as much as you can. Get your proper rest and nutrition and run—but don't forget to take along the ball.

Swimming

TRAINING FOR COMPETITIVE SWIMMING
by Jack Nelson,
Olympic Swimming Coach and Coach of Pinecrest School
and Jack Nelson Swim Club, Fort Lauderdale, Florida

If you want to learn what some of the best young swimmers in the United States are doing today to train for national and world records, then consider these training guidelines. The training program offered here has been tried and tested: it has already produced several Olympic-caliber swimmers and several record-breaking performances. If you want to compete for your school team next season, begin this summer by joining a local swimming club and following the advice of the club's coach. And then pick up my program in September.

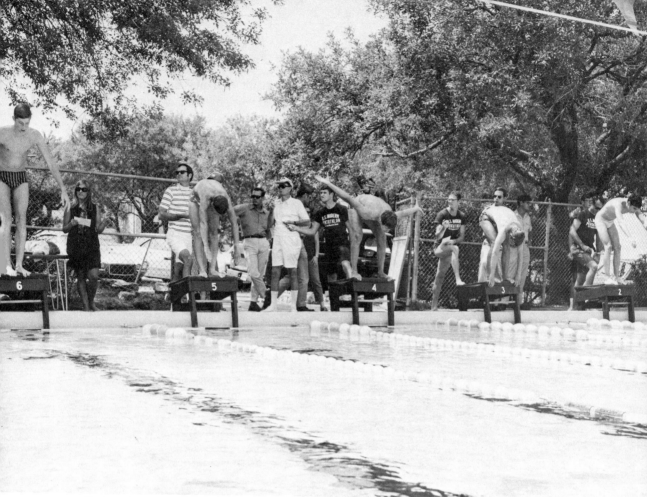

Swimming event at U.S. Olympic Development Clinic Championship. (U.S. Army)

DRY WORKOUTS IN SEPTEMBER

Try the sample morning workout for September, keeping in mind that you are exercising to strengthen and stretch your muscles. The afternoon run as a member of the cross-country team is designed to build your cardio-vascular endurance, that is, increase your heart's and lungs' capacity to deliver oxygen to your muscles.

Work hard on the kangaroo jumps; they are prescribed to build push power off the starting blocks. This early in the season is a good time to watch instructional films on swimming fundamentals. A caution: don't copy someone else's swimming stroke. Develop your own stroke and style by fusing the fundamentals—proper grasping, pulling and pressing of the water—with your natural talent.

The remaining fall months (October and November) should be devoted to pulling, kicking, and paddle-pulling—all overload drills that are designed to prepare you for the quality, or speed work, that leads into the competitive season. Ask your coach to help you train by adjusting your individual goals, if you find that those in the accompanying chart prove too difficult at first.

If this is your first crack at training for competition, try each of the swimming drills at one-half repetitions, which will reduce the total distance by one-half. You should be able to handle these distances without too much trouble. Then, work up to our championship workouts.

Once you enter the competitive season, the long, hard swimming is behind you. From late January through June, which covers both the dual-season meets and championship meets, you should train to maintain your level of fitness and speed. Again, ask your coach to bring you along according to your ability and rate of progress.

DUAL MEETS VERSUS CHAMPIONSHIP MEETS

If you want to become a champion—regional, state or national—you must train *through* your school's dual meets. This means that you cannot direct your training to peak for dual meets. You must compete in them as you encounter them during the competitive schedule, but you must keep your overall program pointed at the championship events which usually occur in the spring months—May and June. Follow this training philosophy and you won't peak too soon, or lose your competitive edge when you really need it.

CONCENTRATION

How do you psych yourself on the starting block? I'm often asked that question and I never directly answer it, because it's not the right question. The question should be: what should you concentrate on when you're on the starting block? And the answer is to think hard about what you're doing and what you're going to do—and nothing else. Not about the swimmer on the next block—he's not going to determine your performance. Not about the crowd—it's not going to move you through the water any faster. When you climb onto the starting block, close out the noise around you and think about what you're going to do when you hit the water.

DEFINITIONS OF TRAINING TERMS

Pulls: Laps in the pool performed with immobilized legs (usually an inner tube wrapped around ankles).

Paddle-pulls: Laps in the pool performed with immobilized legs and flat, plastic paddles strapped to the palms of the hands. These paddles extend about one inch beyond the fingertips and are used to develop proper stroke techniques and muscles in the arms and shoulders.

Kicks: Laps in the pool performed with a styrofoam kick board held to the front with extended arms, which do not stroke or in any way aid in propulsion.

Swim: Normal, unencumbered swimming with legs kicking and hands and arms pulling.

Individual medley: Four different swimming styles—butterfly, backstroke, breaststroke and free style—strung together as one event.

SHAPE UP FOR SPORTS

Streamline locomotive: A drill that features successive fast laps, starting with one and working up to four and then back to one, with one slow lap between each fast set. (See sample workout for November.)

TRAINING PROGRAM

September, October and November: Train to build cardio-vascular endurance and to stretch and strengthen the muscles.

A. Sample Morning Workout, September, 7 A.M. to 7:45 A.M., land exercises:

1. Jumping jacks.
2. Situps.
3. Pushups.
4. Piggybacks (hoist another swimmer on your back and run the length of the gymnasium).
5. Wheelbarrow walks.
6. Giant kangaroo hops (from a standing position, reach down and touch the floor with fingertips, legs bent, and leap forward).
7. Military press.
8. Chinups.

B. Sample Afternoon Workout, September, 3 P.M. to 4:30 P.M.:

Run cross-country, 1½ to 3 miles.

C. Sample Morning Workout, November 7 A.M. to 9 A.M., 30 minutes, land exercises, 1½-hour swim routines:

1. 1,000 yards free-style warm-up.
2. 400 yards individual medley, kick down, swim back.
3. 1,000 yards butterfly.
4. 1,000 yards backstroke.
5. 500 yards breaststroke pull.
6. 500 yards breaststroke swim.
7. 800 yards individual medley swim.
8. 5 x 200 yards free-style kick on 3:30 minutes.

D. Sample Afternoon Workout, November, 3 P.M. to 5 P.M.

1. 500 yards general loosen up. Kick down, swim back, stroke of choice.
2. 12 x 200 yards free style on 1:15 minutes.
   10 x 100 yards butterfly on 1:30 minutes.

      10 x 100 yards backstroke on 1:30 minutes.

      8 x 100 yards breaststroke on 1:40 minutes.

3. 10 x 100 yards individual medley on 1:30 minutes.
4. Streamline locomotive, free style:

    1 length slow, 1 fast.

    1 length slow, 2 fast.

    1 length slow, 3 fast.

    1 length slow, 4 fast.

    1 length slow, 3 fast.

    1 length slow, 2 fast.

    1 length slow, 1 fast.

5. Streamline locomotive, stroke of choice (same sequence as in number 3, butterfly swimmers kick on slow lap).
6. 4 x 500 yards free style on 7:30 minutes.
7. 5 x 100 yards individual medley on 1:30 minutes.

December, January, February: Quality training to increase speed:

A. Sample Morning Workout, December, 7 A.M. to 9 A.M., 15 minutes, land drills for primary swimming muscles (upper body) 1¾ hour swim:

1. Loosen up with 2,000 yards free style.
2. 1,000 yards free-style pull.

    900 yards backstroke pull.

    800 yards butterfly pull.

    800 yards breaststroke pull.

3. 5 x 200 yards free-style paddle-pulls on 3 minutes.
4. 5 x 200 yards free-style paddle-kicks on 2:30 minutes.
5. 1,000 yards free-style swim.

B. Sample Afternoon Workout, December, 3 P.M. to 5 P.M.:

1. Loosen up 400 yards, kick down, swim back, stroke of choice.
2. 5 x 200 butterfly on 3 minutes.

    5 x 200 backstroke on 3 minutes.

    4 x 200 breaststroke on 3:30 minutes.

    7 x 200 free style on 2:30 minutes.

3. 3-men relay races (long-rest repeats).

    Swim 25 yards, rest (teammates swim).

    Swim 50 yards, rest (teammates swim).

    Swim 75 yards, rest (teammates swim).

    Swim 100 yards, rest (teammates swim).

       Swim 75 yards, rest (teammates swim).
       Swim 50 yards, rest (teammates swim).
       Swim 25 yards, rest (teammates swim).
4. 5 x 100 yards individual medley kicks without board on 1:30 minutes.
5. 5 x 50 yards on 1 minute (25 yards over water, any stroke, 25 yards underwater).
6. 10 x 100 yards free style on 2 minutes.
7. 10 x 50 yards butterfly on 1 minute.
     10 x 50 yards backstroke on 1 minute.
     10 x 50 yards breaststroke on 1 minute.
     20 x 50 yards free style on 40 seconds.

March, April, May and June: Train to maintain competitive edge and speed levels.

Tennis

The Stan Smith and Jimmy Connors conditioning programs included here are definitely for the competitive tennis player. These are not the kinds of training routines that you can just jump into. Although the routines themselves are definitely not for the weekend or casual tennis player, it would be well for any tennis player to read this section in order to appreciate the stress that these outstanding players place on conditioning.

YEAR-ROUND TRAINING TIPS
by Stan Smith

OFF-SEASON TRAINING

I recommend two things for the off-season: running long distances and playing other sports. The long distances should be run at a leisurely pace. Two to three miles are sufficient. Play basketball, participate in track and field, ski—keep active in the off-season, even play another racket sport, if that's possible. A word of caution here. Learn the basics of tennis first, if you intend to play other racket sports in the off-season. Retain tennis fundamentals in your muscle memory and then you'll be able to play other racket sports, such as squash and paddle ball, and benefit from the agility and quickness they will demand from you.

PRE-SEASON CONDITIONING

Once the formal tennis practice sessions begin, you might try the following drill, which the Davis Cup team uses:

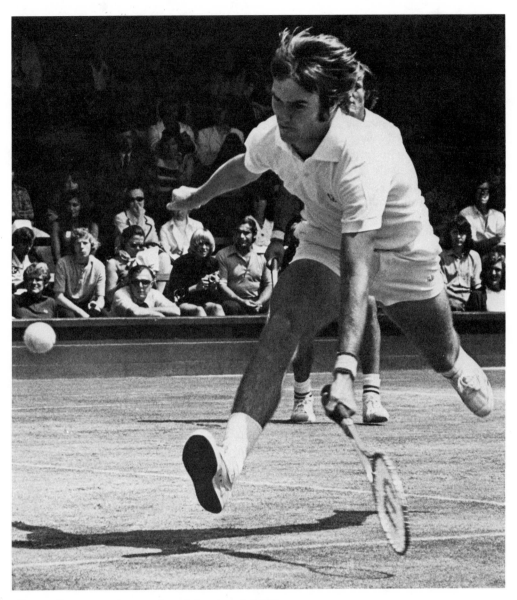

Jimmy Connors returns a tough forehand. (UPI)

12-MINUTE TENNIS CONDITIONING DRILL

Activity	Individual Activity	Cumulative Time
1. Run around outside of courts.	1 min.	1 min.
2. Situps (goal: 1 per sec.).	1 min.	2 min.
3. Run around outside of courts.	1 min.	3 min.
4. Pushups (goals: 20 fingertips in 20 sec.).	20 sec.	3 min., 20 sec.
5. Full arm circles.	40 sec.	4 min.
6. Run around outside of courts.	1 min.	5 min.
7. Squat jumps.	30 sec.	5 min., 30 sec.
8. Toe touches.	30 sec.	6 min.
9. Run around outside of courts.	1 min.	7 min.
10. Hurdler stretches (alternate legs).	1 min.	8 min.
11. Run around outside of courts.	1 min.	9 min.
12. Cross overs (lie on back, arms extended sideward. Touch right foot to left hand, touch left foot to right hand). Side leg raises (lie on side, head resting on right hand. Lift leg high as possible. Repeat opposite leg).	30 sec.	10 min.
13. Run around outside of courts.	1 min.	11 min.
14. Pullups	20 sec.	11 min., 20 sec.
15. Windmill	40 sec.	12 min.
16. Taper off with slow jog around outside of court.		

IN-SEASON DRILLS

You should be in playing shape by this time, so concentrate on improving your timing and quickness. I recommend that you jump rope, run windsprints every other day (40 to 100 yards), and practice your shotmaking ability on the court. Windsprints are extremely important. Because you must continually charge the net in actual matches, you cannot afford to get there slowly, especially late in the matches when a step or two can make the difference between victory and defeat.

DON'T LOSE BECAUSE YOU'RE TIRED
by Jimmy Connors, world's top-rated male tennis player

"Don't let anyone beat you because you're tired." Those are good words of advice from one of tennis' greatest players, Pancho Gonzalez, who first advised me about the importance of conditioning.

If you want to play championship tennis, you have to be in shape. If you're in shape, you know that the only way you can be beaten is if your opponent plays a better match. I've placed Pancho's advice at the top of my list. I stay in shape all-year-round to play tennis.

DAILY ROUTINE

If you want to improve your physical condition for playing tennis, give this daily routine a try. It's worked for me.

Morning Workout

1. Jump rope, 5 to 10 minutes.
2. Jog and run, 1 to 2 miles. Mix up your running by jogging 20 yards, sprinting 20 yards, running backward 20 yards, shuffling sideways for 20 yards and then jogging again.

Afternoon Workout

1. Play 2 to 2½ hours. Play a 2- or 3-set match against a player of equal or superior skill.
2. Practice your shots: Backhands down the line, 5 minutes. Backhands crosscourt, 5 minutes. Forehands down the line, 5 minutes. Forehands crosscourt, 5 minutes. Serves, 5 minutes each court.

2 on 1 Drill

Here is a special drill that will improve not only your cardio-vascular fitness, but also your shotmaking skill. The varsity tennis team at UCLA used to practice this daily and we nicknamed it the "Death Drill" because of its demand on our endurance and stamina. Position two teammates at the net with two dozen balls or more and have them alternate hitting shots to the opposite corners of the baseline. Take a starting position in the middle and begin the drill by running down each shot and hitting them back at your teammates. Continue this drill for 7 or 8 minutes without stopping. Alternate positions at the net with one of your teammates and repeat once more after you have recovered.

HOW TO APPROACH CHALLENGE MATCHES

Any time you're competing for a position on a team, you're going to have to play challenge matches among your teammates to determine who's going to make up the first team. Approach these challenge matches as if you're in an actual tournament. Go in with the attitude that you've got to play just as hard in practice as in actual competition. Get used to playing hard and it will carry over to your tournament matches. In a tournament you only have one chance or you're eliminated. Sharpen your competitive edge in practice; strive to win and never settle for second-best or a half-hearted effort.

PLAY SOCCER TO IMPROVE YOUR FOOTWORK

If you live in a climate that is too cold for tennis in the winter months, take up soccer. I played when I was in high school and found that it not only helped my cardio-vascular endurance, but also improved my agility and balance, skills which helped me play better tennis in the spring. So don't miss an opportunity to improve your footwork when the cold winds blow: play soccer.

TRAINING TECHNIQUE

Here's a training technique that I have found very practical. Seek out the hottest part of the day—even in the summer—and jog easily for 30 to 45 minutes. Sometimes you must play during intense heat, from noon to 3 P.M. and, if you get used to working out in it, it will pay off on the court. Mentally, you'll know the heat cannot get the best of you.

INTENSE EFFORT

I believe that hard work, intense effort, is the secret to improving your tennis. My mother taught me how to play tennis at a very early age. She placed a sawed-off racket in my hand when I was barely able to walk and she guided my practice sessions until age sixteen, when I took instruction from Pancho Gonzalez and Pancho Seguro.

All three of my coaches—Gonzalez, Seguro and my mother—trained me to practice hard and intensely, but not for a long time. I believe that their system—which features brief but intense workouts—helped me to maintain my eagerness and enthusiasm for the game.

Try this approach with your game. Practice the skill you're trying to master as hard and as intensely as possible for a short period of time, perhaps 10 to 15 minutes, and then go on to something else. This method will eliminate sloppy execution—because your muscles will not tire from overexertion—and boredom, because your mind won't have time to meander while you repeatedly "go through the motions."

Wrestling

Wrestling is not your everyday, weekend athlete's cup of tea, but it is a popular scholastic sport at the high school and college levels. Olympic Gold Medal winner Dan Gable describes his warm-up and conditioning programs.

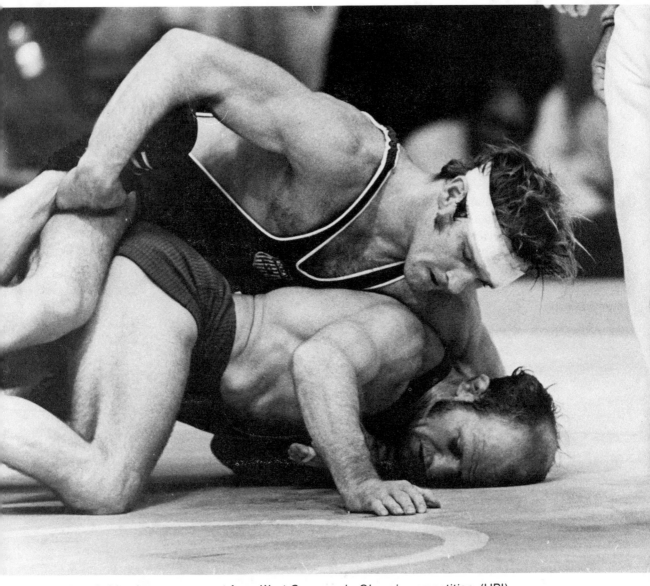

Dan Gable pins an opponent from West Germany in Olympic competition. (UPI)

CONDITIONING FOR WRESTLING
by Dan Gable

THE IMPORTANCE OF PROPER WARM-UP

Once you get into actual competition, one of the most important things to remember is the warm-up. In wrestling, there's always the sudden surprise element and you need to have your body in condition for it. If I'm not thoroughly warm before my match and I go out there and start the match and encounter a surprise move right away, I find myself exhausted and unable to recuperate.

If you're scheduled to wrestle first, you should start warming up before your team gets out there. It's very important before a match to get your body completely loose, every joint and muscle. That way you're going to be relaxed enough not to be injured, and you're going to react better.

Every two minutes or so before my match, I'll get up and do some stretching and limbering exercises—nothing really hard, which could tire you out, but just simple things to get your body loosened up.

When I have time between the weigh-in and the actual competition, sometimes I'll go out and run a mile at a slow pace, get good and loose, then relax. Sprints also help to really get your muscles hot, and flexing exercises get the circulation flowing in your arms and hands.

OFF-SEASON TRAINING PROGRAM FOR WRESTLING
(Off-season spring, summer and fall, if not out for other sports)

I.   Running, 3 times/week (Mon.-Wed.-Fri.).
    A.   Mostly distance (2 miles).
    B.   Sometimes add sprints (100–200 yards, 6–10 reps).

II.   Weight training, 3 times/week (Tues.-Thurs.-Sat.).
    A.   Exercises, sets of 2 or 3:
       1. Curls, reverse curls.
       2. Bench presses.
       3. Rowing.
       4. Tricep extensions.
       5. Squats.
       6. Deltoid, pulling weight from waist to shoulder.
       7. Neck bridging with barbell.

B. Amount of weight—alternate light weight and many repetitions with heavy weight and few repetitions. Ask your coach for minimum pounds to begin with.

III. Wrestling, whenever you can, at least a few times a week.
    A. Drill old and new moves.
    B. Wrestle hard, yet experiment with new things.

IN-SEASON TRAINING PROGRAM FOR WRESTLING

I. Before-school workout (vary from time to time, 45–60 minutes).
    A. Running in gym or outside (weather permitting):
        1. Distance, 10–20 minutes.
        2. Sprints, 10–20 reps gym distance.
    B. Muscle exercises (no limit to reps. Exercise until fatigued):
        1. Pushups, 3 sets.
        2. Chinups, 3 sets.
        3. Situps, 3 sets.
    C. Jumping rope.

II. Wrestling practice (1½ to 2 hours).
    A. Coaches' actual time:
        1. Always be on time.
        2. Work harder than anyone else.
        3. Never leave until fatigued.
    B. Wrestler's own time:
        1. Drill moves.
        2. Wrestle combatively (conditioning).

III. Directly after wrestling practice (3–4 times/week, 20 minutes).
    A. Muscle exercises (pushups, chinups, situps—3 sets each).
    B. Weight training (2–3 sets each):
        1. Curls.
        2. Tricep extensions overhead.
        3. Rowing with barbell or dumbbell.
        4. Squats, or any thigh exercise.
        5. Deltoids, pull weight from waist to shoulder.
    C. Amount of weight—enough weight so only 8–12 reps can be completed.

Note: The pace should increase in everything above as the season progresses toward the tournaments. If time does not permit you to work out this much, remember the most important thing in winning: wrestle hard during the coaches' actual practice time.

GENERAL TIPS TO HELP YOU SUCCEED IN WRESTLING

1. *Wrestle longer than the normal time period.* Often the best way to learn is not to have a clock over your head telling you to hurry up. You need time to experiment, realize what you're trying to work on and figure out how to improve.

2. *Vary your workouts to avoid monotony.* I try to get a different schedule all the time, and make a game out of my exercises. Often, when I run, I'll have a friend drive alongside in his car with the window down and music playing on the radio. It helps keep my mind off running. Or, in curls with weights, I'll get a buddy and I'll do one curl and hand it to him and he does one; then he hands it to me and I do two; then he does two, and so on up the line until we're each doing ten repetitions without ever setting the weight down. We try to do the curls as strictly as possible, and it really builds our endurance. But without the buddy I wouldn't be able to push myself that hard.

3. *Work all-year-round.* I've found that conditioning for a one-season sport can be pretty bad, if you just let that season be your season. Every sport offered in high school can help you improve your wrestling, at the same time giving you some variety. Football will toughen you up, track will help your endurance and sports like tennis and baseball will teach you coordination and quick reactions.

4. *Learn how to practice on your own.* It may be fun to work with a buddy sometimes, but I know I've learned as much in wrestling from doing things by myself as I have with other people. You have to learn the technique. Your coach can show you the right steps to take in a fireman's carry, for instance, and you can walk through these yourself in your basement or out on the grass. Another thing I've done is to borrow a football dummy and use it like an opponent to practice my steps or how to use my legs in a certain situation.

5. *Don't starve yourself.* Cutting out food and water takes a lot of fight out of you and will hinder your performance. It's better to eat small meals two or three times a day than to have just one big meal. You'll have more energy for practice and you'll also shrink your stomach so you'll never have to eat a lot to feel full.